the 30-DAY
THYROID RESET PLAN

PAGE STREET
PUBLISHING CO.

Copyright © 2018 Becky Campbell

First published in 2018 by
Page Street Publishing Co.
27 Congress Street, Suite 105
Salem, MA 01970
www.pagestreetpublishing.com

Distributed by Macmillan, sales in Canada by The Canadian Manda Group.

This book is intended to supplement, not replace, the advice of a trained health professional. If you know or suspect that you have a health problem, you should consult a health professional. In addition, if you have any questions or uncertainty about implementing anything in this book, you should consult a health professional.

23 22 21 20 19   3 4 5 6 7

ISBN-13: 978-1-62414-571-1
ISBN-10: 1-62414-571-X

Library of Congress Control Number: 2017952268

Cover and book design by Page Street Publishing Co.
Photography by Toni Zernik and Lindsey Potter

Printed and bound in the United States

the 30-DAY THYROID RESET PLAN

DISARMING THE 7 HIDDEN TRIGGERS
THAT ARE KEEPING YOU SICK

DR. BECKY CAMPBELL

Foreword by Chris Kresser, M.S., LAc

PAGE STREET
PUBLISHING CO.

contents

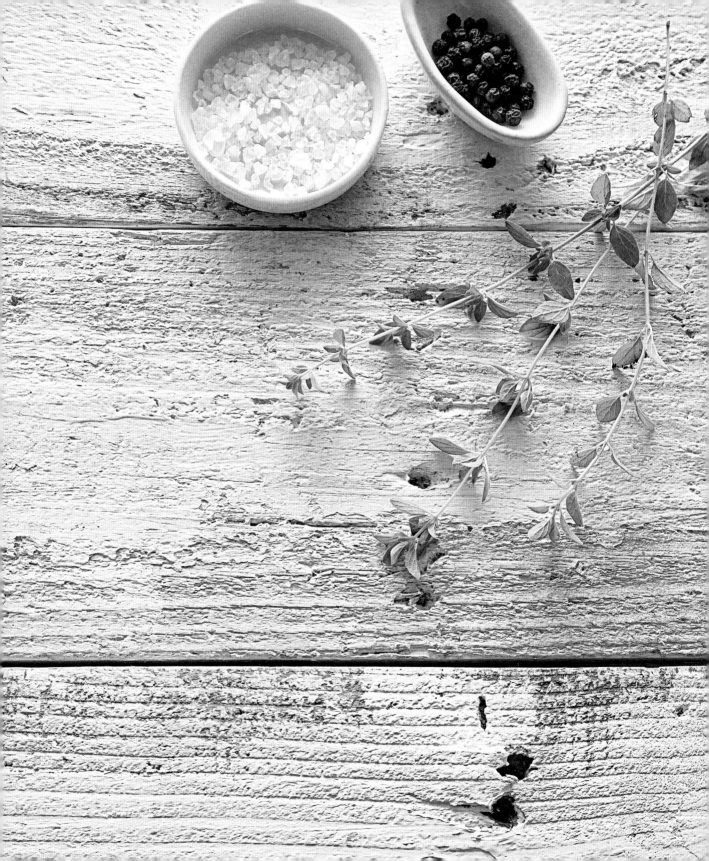

FOREWORD

—

"So what is disease? In old times people used to think that a disease was some actual entity or thing which had got into the body in some way, and was there lying hidden and secreted, and was to be cast out. This idea, which we now know to be true only in a few specific instances, was at one time general. ... The conclusion is that all disease is disordered function. Here, then, I say, is the highest justification for all treatment being based upon the principle of restoring disordered functions to order, and this is what I have ventured to term Functional Medicine."

—**WILLOUGHBY F. WADE,** BA, MB, Physician to the General Hospital, Birmingham, England
Delivered as a Clinical Lecture on Functional Medicine, March 5, 1870
Published in the July 1, 1871 issue of *The Lancet*

If you follow popular media, you might think that the greatest threat to human health is infectious disease. In the summer of 2016, it was impossible to open a newspaper or web browser without seeing headlines like this:

"Deadly disease spread by mosquitoes could kill MILLIONS in plague-like global pandemic, world's richest man Bill Gates warns"

"Mosquito-borne pandemic could wipe out 10 million people"

"Zika—a threat bigger than World War"

It's hard not to feel worried by headlines like this. Yet although Zika has potentially serious complications, including birth defects and (rarely) death, in 2016 the WHO estimated that only three to four million people worldwide would contract the disease, and most would not show any symptoms.

If acute infections like Zika aren't the primary threat to human health, what is? Consider the following:

- Globally, chronic disease is responsible for twice as many deaths as infectious disease.
- One in two Americans now has a chronic disease; one in four Americans have more than one chronic disease.
- In 1994, 13 percent of children had a chronic disease—it has now more than doubled to 27 percent.
- The number of chronic disease diagnoses is expected to increase by 42 percent in the next 15 years.
- Of the $3.2 trillion we spend on health care in the United States, 86 percent goes toward treating chronic disease.
- Chronic disease will account for $47 trillion in health care expenditure by 2030 if the epidemic is unchecked. That's more than the annual gross domestic product (GDP) of the six largest economies in the world.

Given these statistics, it should be clear that chronic illness—not infectious disease—is our biggest health care challenge. It's an unnatural, slow-motion plague that is destroying our quality of life, bankrupting our economies, and threatening the health of future generations. And although it's unfolding over a longer time scale, it is arguably just as much of a threat to our civilization and way of life as the bubonic plague was to Europe in the fourteenth century.

Chronic disease is now so common that we think it's normal. But there's a big difference between what's common, and what's normal. Contrary to what current statistics may suggest, it is *not* normal for human beings to develop chronic illness.

Studies of contemporary hunter-gatherer populations that have retained their traditional diet and lifestyle suggest that they are remarkably lean and fit and superior to people living in the industrialized world in almost every measure of health and fitness, including body mass index, blood pressure, vision, bone density, and cardiovascular function.

Some believe that hunter-gatherers don't develop chronic disease because they don't live long enough to acquire it. It's true that our ancestors had shorter life spans than ours. These averages, however, don't account for the high rates of death from violence, warfare, exposure to the elements, acute infections, and sepsis. Research has shown that when hunter-gatherers have access to even the most rudimentary forms of emergency medical care, they live life spans equivalent to ours today—but they reach old age without acquiring the chronic, debilitating diseases that characterize our senior years and, increasingly, even our younger years.

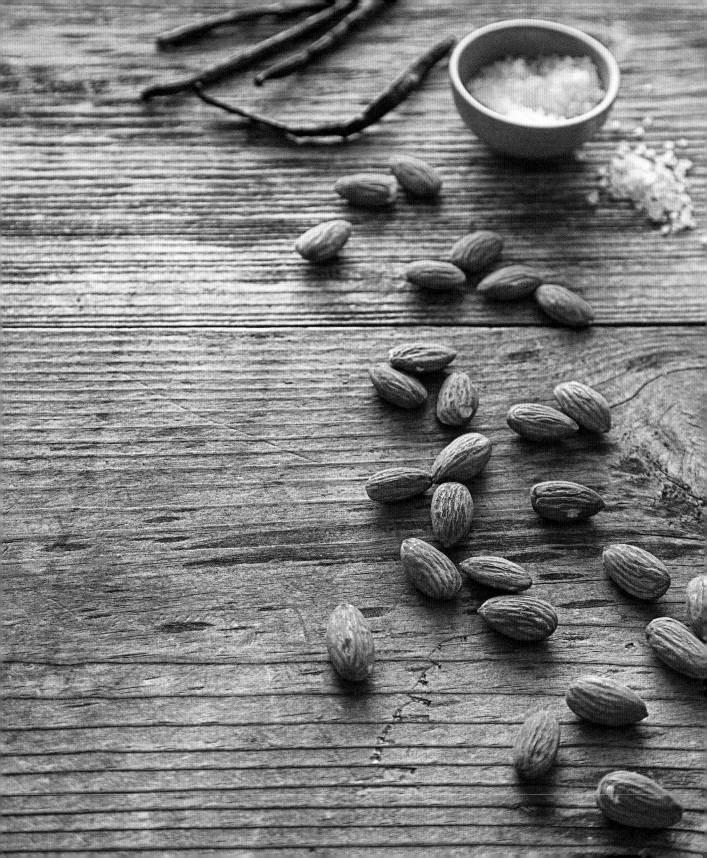

It's not only our hunter-gatherer ancestors who experienced lower rates of chronic disease; even our grandparents and great-grandparents were significantly healthier than we are today. For example, the Centers for Disease Control estimates that obesity rates in the United States have increased by a whopping 185 percent over the last 50 years. American adults saw their rate of obesity jump from 13 percent of the population in 1960 to more than 38 percent in 2014. The increase of obesity in children has been even more dramatic: from just 5 percent to more than 17 percent, a jump of over 230 percent. These are profound changes in just two generations.

What happened? Why has chronic disease exploded so dramatically over the past several decades, with apparently no end in sight? There are many reasons, but one of the most significant is that our medical model is simply not set up to adequately address chronic health problems.

Our current medical paradigm evolved during a time when acute, infectious disease was the biggest threat to our health. In 1900 the top causes of death were typhoid, tuberculosis, and pneumonia. Other reasons that people visited the doctor also tended to be acute, such as a gallbladder attack or appendicitis. Treatment was relatively straightforward: The doctor gave an antibiotic (once they were invented), or the surgeon removed the gallbladder or appendix, and the patient got better. One problem, one doctor, one treatment.

Today, however, seven of the top ten causes of death are chronic, rather than acute, diseases. Chronic diseases are difficult to manage, expensive to treat, and usually last a lifetime. They don't lend themselves to the "one problem, one doctor, one treatment" model of the past. Today's patient has multiple diseases, sees multiple doctors (a different one for every part of the body, in fact), and requires multiple treatments.

Conventional medicine simply isn't set up to treat today's patients. We desperately need a new approach—one that is focused not on simply suppressing symptoms with drugs and surgery, but on addressing the underlying causes of chronic disease.

Fortunately, such an approach already exists, and it's called functional medicine. Functional medicine is different than conventional medicine in several ways:

- It treats symptoms by addressing the root causes of the problem.
- It views the body as an interconnected, biological ecosystem rather than just a collection of separate parts.
- It relies primarily on diet, lifestyle, and behavior change, along with supplements and botanicals, rather than drugs.
- It recognizes the individuality of the patient and acknowledges that there's no one-size-fits-all approach.
- It empowers the patient to play an active role in his or her healing process.

If you haven't yet heard of functional medicine, you will soon. Cleveland Clinic, one of the most prestigious medical institutions in the world, has invested tens of millions in a new Center for Functional Medicine, spearheaded by Dr. Mark Hyman. Primary care groups like Intermountain and Iora Health have incorporated functional medicine principles into their care models, and are saving thousands of dollars a year and improving the lives of countless patients.

Many clinicians, myself included, firmly believe that it represents the future of medicine and is the only hope we have of reversing the chronic disease epidemic. That is why I've spent the last several years training nearly 400 clinicians around the world in a functional medicine approach to treating (and preventing) chronic disease.

In this book, *The 30-Day Thyroid Reset Plan*, Dr. Becky Campbell applies a functional medicine framework to addressing thyroid disorders. Dr. Campbell struggled with an undiagnosed thyroid condition for many years, and it wasn't until she discovered functional medicine that she was able to successfully treat it and restore her health. This experience inspired her to pursue training in functional medicine, and she was one of the first graduates of the Kresser Institute ADAPT Framework Functional Medicine Training Program.

Like most chronic diseases, thyroid disorders are poorly treated by conventional medicine. The typical approach is based on the replacement model: If thyroid hormone levels are low, the doctor simply prescribes synthetic (or in some cases, natural) thyroid hormone medication. Although this can be effective, and is sometimes necessary, it doesn't address the root causes of poor thyroid function, which include autoimmunity, nutrient deficiency, inflammation, gut dysfunction, chronic stress, and environmental toxins. This means that the patient will have to take thyroid hormones for the rest of her life, often at higher and higher doses, as the underlying problems continue to go unaddressed.

Fortunately, the functional medicine approach to treating thyroid problems that Dr. Campbell will share with you in this book offers you the opportunity to truly heal your condition. And although thyroid hormone replacement may still be required in some cases, most patients will be able to get by with a lower dose after addressing the root causes of their thyroid problem. In many other cases, patients will be able to avoid—or even stop—taking thyroid medication altogether.

This inside-out healing, using natural remedies like diet and lifestyle, is the promise of this book you're holding in your hands now, and of functional medicine in general. Congratulations for taking a huge leap toward greater control over your health, and a longer, disease-free life!

—CHRIS KRESSER, MS, LAC

Founder, Kresser Institute and ChrisKresser.com
Co-Founder and President, California Center for Functional Medicine

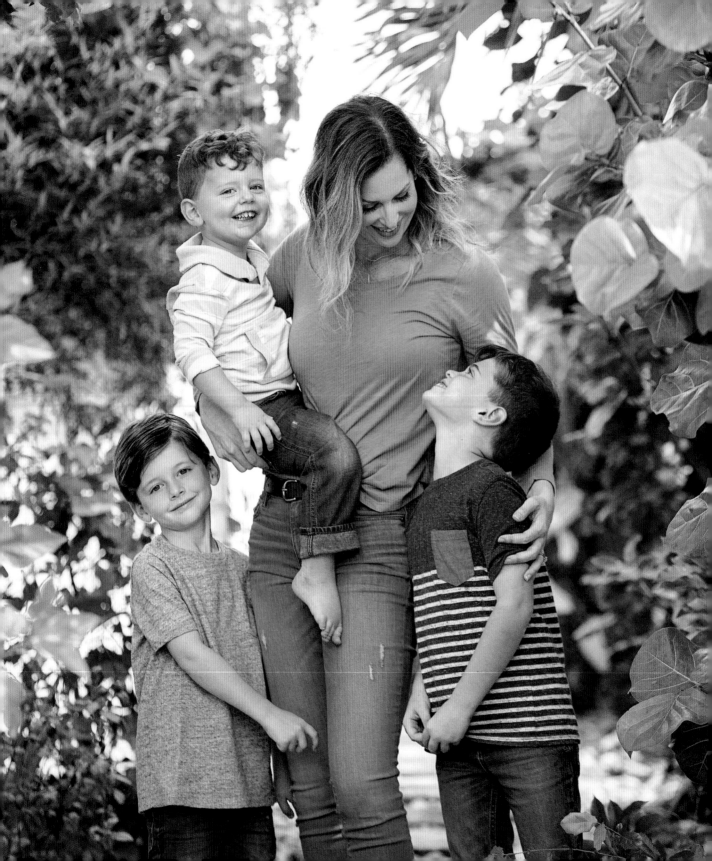

INTRODUCTION

If you're reading this book, the very first thing I want you to know before you turn another page is that you are not alone in how you feel. How do I know this? I know this because my start in functional medicine all began with my own health crisis starting as far back as high school, and I see patients in my practice dealing with very similar issues you may be suffering from today.

Before you dive into this book, I want to share my personal story with you. I want you to know that I'm not just the standard functional medicine practitioner. I am a practitioner who has been in your shoes and has been down the modern medical route time and time again with disappointment. This is why I am passionate about what I do, because I can relate to almost every one of my patients on a personal level. I know how hard it is to be sick and tired of feeling sick and tired and feeling like no doctor can give you an answer. This is why it's my mission to help patients uncover their own personal root cause each day I show up to work. So here is my story, and how I went from being sick to finding my root cause and eventually putting all of my symptoms into remission. I believe that it sets the tone for the book—that there is hope and that feeling better is possible. I offer this inspiration to help you move forward toward uncovering root causes and to keep advocating for your health.

For as long as I can remember, I have never felt good. I remember being younger and wanting to go home from school because I was tired or just didn't feel well. In high school, I missed a lot of my early morning classes because I couldn't get out of bed on time. I remember being so fatigued, and it seemed like I was the only one that was dealing with this. No one else around me seemed to have any of the same issues. While I was trying to get through high school, I was also trying to figure out why I felt so exhausted all of the time.

Fast-forward to college when I started to learn how to take better care of myself. I was eating a very clean diet for the most part, and I was exercising six days a week. I was in excellent shape. I had always been on the thin side, but I was now really toned as well. This was probably the best I had felt my whole life. This lasted for a couple of years. Then suddenly those draining symptoms from the previous years were back, but it was way worse than before. The weight gain came on suddenly; in fact, I gained 30 pounds (13 kg) out of nowhere. I was so fatigued that I could barely stay awake, and I had a severe case of brain fog. I felt like I was walking around in a dream. I also started to suffer from severe anxiety and panic attacks. Not only had I gained weight, but I was getting so bloated after I ate. I felt like I looked six months pregnant! I remember being at work and thinking that if I could just take two-minute naps all day, I could make it through. This was not good; I could not go on living my life like this, and I had to figure out what was wrong.

I started to go to different doctors, one after the other, and they all looked at me like I was crazy. Since my blood panel was coming back "normal," they told me I was fine and tried to put me on anti-anxiety and anti-depression medication. I wasn't depressed, I was sick, and no one knew what was wrong, and I felt like no one believed me. I was put on a number of ridiculous medications that only made me feel worse.

Finally, I learned about functional medicine and found a practitioner that I hoped could help me. They ran tests that were far different than any I had ever had before. They did a stool test to look for infections in my gut, they did a saliva test to look for adrenal gland dysfunction, and they looked at my blood panel using functional medicine ranges instead of the conventional medicine ranges. (You will learn the importance of these lab ranges throughout the book.) These tests were far more comprehensive and thorough than what my other physicians were willing to run. When I got the results back, it turned out that I had candida, parasites, high cortisol levels, the Epstein-Barr virus, and many food intolerances. I also had an issue with my thyroid that no one ever found before because they were going by the conventional medicine ranges that are way too broad, which I now know is one of the leading causes of thyroid misdiagnoses. I was also diagnosed with hypoglycemia (low blood sugar), which was triggering my anxiety and panic attacks.

I went through treatment for all of these things, and it completely changed my life. I immediately lost the 30 pounds I had gained, plus more, I had a lot more energy, and my brain fog was gone. After I went through treatment, I felt amazing, and I knew that I wanted to help people find the underlying causes of their symptoms and disease. This is what sparked my interest and passion for working in the functional medicine field. There are so many people dealing with the exact or a very similar situation that I went through for years. Being misdiagnosed, overprescribed, and even misprescribed medications because the root cause is not uncovered. Being looked at as crazy or having anxiety or depression just because a doctor cannot put their finger on what's causing your symptoms. I went through this, and I know that there are thousands of people who are dealing with this exact situation today.

Since I began my journey working with functional medicine practitioners years ago, I have continued to feel better every single day since I uncovered my root cause, but I still suffered from mild fatigue. However, once I learned how to practice functional medicine myself, I figured out that I also had mercury toxicity, leaky gut, and mast cell activation syndrome. I have learned how to put all of this into remission and how to keep it that way.

My goal in sharing my personal story with you and in writing this book is to help you understand that there are underlying causes of your symptoms. It is not usually just one thing, it can be many things, and we can figure out what they are and what to do about them so that you can live an abundant and healthy life free from debilitating symptoms.

WHAT IF YOUR DOCTOR WON'T TAKE YOUR SYMPTOMS SERIOUSLY?

Chances are, if you have picked up this book, you may be looking for a different approach to modern-day medicine. One of the many reasons patients end up searching for a functional medicine practitioner is because their doctors just aren't taking their symptoms seriously. I have been there and done that. Since my lab values were normal, I was also one of the patients who was told that I should just go on anti-anxiety and anti-depression medication. The problem is that that's not what was going on in my body at all. I had some serious imbalances that were causing me to feel the way that I did. The issue was that I wasn't seeing the right doctors. I wasn't seeing physicians who were willing to take a really good hard look at what was going on.

Unfortunately, in today's medical field, many practitioners aren't looking past lab values for a diagnosis, and this is not to mention that mainstream medicine doesn't look at functional lab ranges. You will learn more about this in the coming chapters. If you are reading this book today and feel like your doctor just will not take your symptoms seriously and that you have been to doctor after doctor looking for answers, please know that you are not alone! So many of my patients come to me after suffering from exhaustion, weight gain, hair loss, depression, pain, and other debilitating symptoms for years. Many of these patients have not yet received the proper testing that they need to find out what is really going on and causing all of those symptoms they have been living with for years. I always tell my patients that you know your body best, and you know when something is not right. The sad reality is that often times when doctors don't know what is wrong with you, they will tell you it's all in your head and will try to prescribe psychiatric medications just as they did in my situation.

If you are fed up with feeling like you can't find a doctor who takes your symptoms seriously, I want to congratulate you for picking up this book and reading it. This is a massive step in advocating for yourself and for your health.

Throughout this book, I am going to walk you through steps you can take to uncover what your root cause may be and to help you start to feel better by taking the steps you need to balance your overall health. I will also walk you through some of the testing that is offered through functional medicine that can assist you in getting to the bottom of what is going on with your health.

If you are new to functional medicine, head over to the next section where I talk about the differences between a functional medicine approach and conventional medicine.

Again, congratulations for taking this journey today! You are one step closer to uncovering your root cause and getting on a healthier track advocating for your own health throughout the whole process.

THE FUNCTIONAL MEDICINE APPROACH

What is functional medicine? To help you understand what a functional medicine approach is, I want to first break down the biggest difference between this approach to health and a conventional approach to health.

When talking about conventional medicine, the focus is more on pathology. It's looking for disease. In functional medicine, we look to see where the problem is coming from before it turns into disease. If you come to a functional medicine practitioner when you have already been diagnosed, a functional medicine approach can work to help keep that disease at bay with the ultimate goal of helping you get your life back.

To further elaborate on functional medicine, here are some ways I like to define it. Functional medicine is:

- INVESTIGATIVE. Addresses symptoms by focusing on the underlying cause of the problem, which leads to more profound and longer lasting results.

- HOLISTIC. Envisions the body as an interconnected whole that is in dynamic relationship to its environment, and recognizes the importance of these connections in health and disease.

- SAFE. Has mild or no side effects, and other unrelated complaints often improve spontaneously.

- PATIENT-CENTERED. Treats the patient, not the disease. Treatments are highly individualized based on patient needs.

- PARTICIPATORY. Respects, empowers, and educates patients. Patients are encouraged to play an active role in the healing process.

- INTEGRATIVE. Combines the best of both modern and traditional medicines and emphasizes importance of diet and lifestyle.

- RESTORATIVE. Designs tests and treatments to promote optimal function, prevent and reverse disease, and improve quality of life.

- PREVENTATIVE. Draws wisdom from the ancient Chinese saying, "The superb physician treats disease before it occurs."

- EVIDENCE-BASED. Uses the latest research from peer-reviewed medical journals and is uncorrupted by corporate and political interests.

So many of the patients that I see have gone down the modern medical route of seeing dozens of doctors. They have been through numerous different studies and tests, and are taking a handful of medications. However, the problem is that many of these patients have seen very minimal results, and some haven't even had any relief at all.

If you are looking to take an investigative, safe, and holistic approach to your health, then functional medicine may be for you! Reading this book is your first step in understanding the cause of your symptoms, so that you may not have to rely on medications or other interventions for the rest of your life. Even if medication is necessary for your situation, a functional medicine approach always allows for active participation in one's life and one's health, which is incredibly empowering and rewarding.

Functional medicine is all about helping you live your life to the fullest, helping you unmask your symptoms, and getting you on a healthier path long-term. While this book focuses on Hashimoto's thyroiditis and other thyroid conditions, keep in mind that functional medicine is used to treat a wide variety of conditions and can help you in more than just one area of your health. Remember, it's a well-rounded, holistic approach to health, so whether you are trying to boost thyroid health or live a healthier lifestyle all around, functional medicine may be the option for you.

I chose to write this book on thyroid health because of the battle I went through. I felt terrible for many years, had a handful of different symptoms, and had health conditions that all led to a thyroid condition. Unfortunately, no one was able to diagnose my thyroid condition for many years. It took uncovering my root cause to get to the bottom of what triggered my thyroid condition. Through my own struggles came my passion for helping others dealing with the same frustrating battle of being misdiagnosed or having their symptoms overlooked.

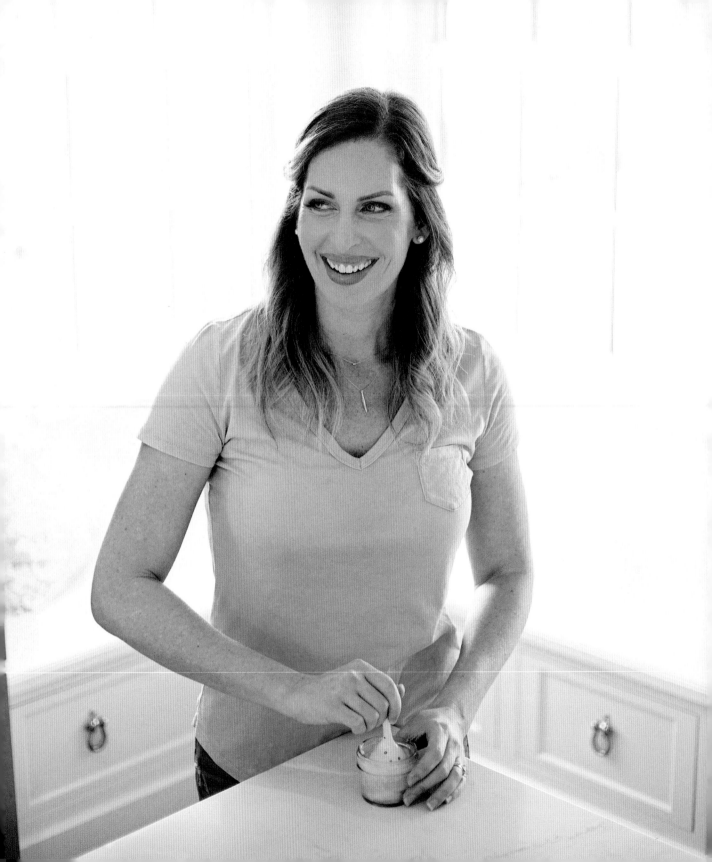

one

AN INTRODUCTION TO
THE THYROID

Thyroid conditions are something that many Americans suffer from. In fact, it is estimated that 20 million Americans have some form of thyroid disease and nearly 60 percent of those with a thyroid condition are not even aware that they have one according to the American Thyroid Association. Here is just one reason why it's so important to understand how our thyroid functions. Why is our thyroid important and what does it do? Let's dive deeper into that.

You have probably been told that the thyroid is a butterfly-shaped gland, that it is part of the endocrine system, and that it is located at the base of the neck, but what about what the thyroid does? The thyroid plays a very important role in metabolism. It's responsible for releasing hormones that control the metabolism, which is the way that the body uses energy. Not only that, but the thyroid controls a number of other bodily functions through producing, storing, and releasing hormones into our bloodstream.

Here are some of the body functions the thyroid controls:

- Heart rate
- Breathing
- The central and peripheral nervous system
- Weight

- Menstrual cycles
- Muscle strength
- Body temperature
- Cholesterol

These hormones then enter into our body's cells. The thyroid uses the iodine we consume from foods to create the two primary thyroid hormones: triiodothyronine (T3) and thyroxine (T4). For optimal health, these two hormones must be carefully balanced. It is critical that T3 and T4 do not become too high or too low. So, what controls this balance? The hypothalamus and the pituitary gland, two glands located in the brain, communicate with one another to help keep these two hormones in check. The hypothalamus produces thyrotropin-releasing hormone, which in turn stimulates the release of thyroid-stimulating hormone (TSH), which then alerts the pituitary gland to let the thyroid know it should be making either more or less T3 and T4. This is done by increasing or decreasing thyroid-stimulating hormone. For example, when T3 and T4 levels are too low, more TSH will be released to alert the thyroid that it needs to make more thyroid hormones.

This can seem complicated, and it truly is an intricate and delicate balance, but don't worry about memorizing exactly how your thyroid works. Just know that an imbalance in T3 or T4 can cause a thyroid imbalance and that your thyroid is in charge of maintaining the balance of a number of different body processes. Without your thyroid, your health would suffer in more ways than one. T3 and T4 reach nearly every cell in the body and regulate things like heart rate as well as metabolism and how quickly your intestines process food. With an imbalance, your heart rate could be too fast or too slow, you could have joint pain or heavy periods, or you could suffer from constipation or diarrhea.

Let's take a look at what happens to the body when there is an imbalance in thyroid hormones. This will give you a clearer picture as to just how important thyroid hormone levels are and why your symptoms may appear to be very random and affect nearly every part of your body.

TOO LITTLE T3 AND T4 IN THE BODY

Hypothyroidism (*hypo* means "below") is too little T3 and T4 present. Symptoms include:

- Fatigue
- Dry skin
- Depression

- Sensitivity to cold
- Joint and/or muscle pain
- Heavy periods

TOO MUCH T3 AND T4 IN THE BODY

Hyperthyroidism (*hyper* means "over") is too much T3 and T4 present. Symptoms include:

- Hair loss
- Absent or light menstrual cycles
- Anxiety

- Nervousness
- Shakiness
- Irritability

THE THYROID AND THE BODY'S SYSTEMS

Thyroid disease affects every part of the body. The following is an overview of its effects on the various systems.

CARDIOVASCULAR SYSTEM

As previously mentioned, heart rate can be affected by changes in thyroid hormones, and the rest of the cardiovascular system can be affected as well. In cases where there is too much thyroid hormone (hyperthyroidism), you may notice a faster heart rate, higher blood pressure, and lower exercise performance. In cases where there is too little thyroid hormone (hypothyroidism), there is often a slower heart rate and lower blood pressure. With hypothyroidism, there is also a higher risk of atherosclerosis as well as heart attack, which is why it is so important to get your thyroid health under control as soon as possible.

Anemia is also something that can result from Hashimoto's thyroiditis. In fact, people with Hashimoto's disease are more likely to develop other autoimmune conditions, including pernicious anemia. Pernicious anemia is caused by not having enough B12 in the body. When anemia is present, the number of red blood cells is lower than normal, which can ultimately lead to less oxygen transport to body cells and cause terrible fatigue.

DIGESTIVE SYSTEM

Another common symptom of hypothyroidism is constipation, while the opposite is true for hyperthyroidism. When dealing with a thyroid condition, your metabolism is altered, which is one of the reasons your digestive system is affected. In cases of hypothyroidism, stomach acid production may be halted as hypothyroidism commonly affects the hormone gastrin. When there's not sufficient gastrin being produced, there's not enough stomach acid, which can lead to symptoms like heartburn because too little stomach acid is as problematic as too much stomach acid. We need stomach acid for proper digestion, and so, without enough, digestion will be compromised.

Malabsorption can also result from thyroid disease. Malabsorption occurs when the small intestine does not absorb the vitamins and minerals from the foods we eat. Malabsorption of vitamin B12, which can ultimately lead to anemia, is an example.

Another common issue with the thyroid and digestive connection is food allergies and sensitivities. Most people with autoimmune conditions also suffer from leaky gut, so focusing on gut health is a crucial step in addressing thyroid health as well. Diet choices are also incredibly important. If you are consuming inflammatory or reactive foods, you could be doing daily harm to your overall health. Addressing all of this at its root is a huge step in getting onto a path of remission.

NERVOUS SYSTEM

The central nervous system can be affected by either too little or too much thyroid hormone. A common symptom of hypothyroidism is brain fog—the feeling of being slightly disconnected or unable to think clearly. This is due to the lack of thyroid hormones circulating that in turn affects the central nervous system. Depression is also a common symptom of hypothyroidism. Too much thyroid hormone also affects the central nervous system, typically in the form of anxiety or excessive irritability.

The central nervous system is impacted so significantly by our thyroid hormones that recent studies have come out stating that hypothyroidism and Hashimoto's disease are linked to the development of Alzheimer's, Parkinson's, and Huntington's disease. This just proves the effect thyroid hormones play in every aspect of our health, including our brain.

REPRODUCTIVE SYSTEM

Many women who suffer from thyroid conditions also suffer from reproductive issues. Hypothyroidism is often linked with heavy periods and even infertility. One of the reasons for this is that hypothyroidism can cause a reduction in progesterone. Not having enough progesterone affects the menstrual cycle.

ADRENAL GLANDS

Adrenal health and thyroid health are truly intertwined. The adrenal glands produce and secrete numerous hormones. Stress plays an important role in the health of our adrenal glands and can throw our hormones out of whack. With chronic stress, the body can eventually get to the point where the adrenal glands are not producing enough, which is called adrenal fatigue.

Adrenal fatigue occurs in different stages. You may start out dealing with a stressor, such as a job interview. Your body makes the hormones that it needs in order to properly respond to this stress—cortisol and epinephrine, which you likely know as adrenaline. The next stage is when this stress doesn't go away—you get the job, but your boss is difficult, the commute is long, and you have many new responsibilities. As the stress continues, your body continues to react to it.

Your adrenal glands will start to become stressed if you are not dealing with all the new stressors in a healthy way. You may begin to notice symptoms, like feeling wired at certain points of the day, and then exhausted at others. The next stage is when adrenal-produced hormones like DHEA (dehydroepiandrosterone) start to drop. You may notice you feel tired and are getting sick more often. This stage can occur for a long time, and in some people it lasts for years. Finally is the phase where your body stops effectively producing hormones. Not only is cortisol low, but other sex hormones are at an all-time low as well. This is when adrenal fatigue kicks in and you may notice irritability, anxiety, weight loss, and chronic fatigue.

So how are the adrenals linked to thyroid health? Having adrenal fatigue puts you at a greater risk of losing sensitivity to thyroid hormones. Having adrenal fatigue can also cause your body to decrease the conversion of T4 to T3 in usable form, can disrupt the immune system barriers in the body, and can even prevent the thyroid hormones from being absorbed into the cells of the body.

WHAT IS AN AUTOIMMUNE DISEASE?

Now that you know the function of your thyroid, it's important to talk about autoimmune diseases. Autoimmune diseases may affect nearly 50 million Americans, according to the American Autoimmune Related Diseases Association (AARDA).

An autoimmune disease occurs when your immune system attacks healthy cells. Your immune system is responsible for defending your body against harmful disease, but with autoimmune conditions, your immune system is hypersensitive and starts going after your body's cells. This can occur anywhere in the body—the thyroid, kidneys, or gastrointestinal tract, for example. Depending on what autoimmune condition is present, the disease could even attack more than one area at a time, while also causing changes in organ function.

Autoimmune diseases are so difficult to diagnose because there are at least 80 different types, many of them have similar symptoms, and it's even possible to have more than one at one time. These diseases can also go into remission for periods of time, making diagnosis more of a challenge. While there is no cure for autoimmune diseases, there is a lot you can do with dietary, supplemental, and lifestyle changes to send the disease into remission and maintain remission. It's about getting to the root cause, identifying triggers, and keeping triggers to a minimum to allow the body to heal and stay in remission for longer periods of time.

THE DIFFERENT TYPES OF THYROID DISEASES

HYPERTHYROIDISM: When the thyroid produces too much thyroid hormone, it is referred to as hyperthyroidism. In this condition, the thyroid is overactive.

GRAVES' DISEASE: Graves' disease is the most common cause of hyperthyroidism. Graves' disease is an autoimmune condition where the thyroid produces too much thyroid hormone. While the actual cause of this autoimmune disease is unknown, it's thought that this condition often runs in families, so you could be genetically predisposed if a family member suffers from this condition. You may also be more likely to develop this autoimmune condition if you suffer from poor gut health or any one of the seven triggers we will be focusing on in this book. So, what happens when you have Graves' disease? Your immune system starts to create antibodies that will trigger the thyroid to make more thyroid hormone than it needs. Some of the symptoms of Graves' disease include anxiety, weight loss, insomnia, chest pain and/or palpitations, shortness of breath, increased bowel movements, goiter, irregular menstrual periods, and vision problems.

HYPOTHYROIDISM: Hypothyroidism is an underactive thyroid gland. This is a condition where the thyroid gland does not make enough thyroid hormone and therefore there is not enough thyroid hormone in the blood. There are different causes of hypothyroidism, but Hashimoto's thyroiditis, a pituitary disorder where the pituitary gland does not make enough TSH, is the most common cause. Hypothyroidism can occur during or after pregnancy, as a result of thyroid damage from radiation treatment, or as a side effect of some medications.

HASHIMOTO'S THYROIDITIS: Hashimoto's thyroiditis is the most common thyroid condition in the United States today and affects nearly 14 million people. Treating Hashimoto's is what I specialize in, which is why this thyroid condition is the focus of this book. Do keep in mind that all of this information in this book is valuable for any type of health condition, as it's all about a holistic approach to health.

As you now know, an autoimmune disease is when the body starts to attack its own tissue. In Hashimoto's thyroiditis, the body attacks the thyroid by marking the thyroid as foreign. The attack on the thyroid leads to a depletion of T4 and T3 or can even go on to completely destroy the thyroid. This can ultimately lead to hypothyroidism, which is when the thyroid does not produce enough hormones and can lead to the need for additional medication. Hashimoto's thyroiditis may be caused by genetic, dietary, hormonal, or environmental factors.

One of the most common signs of this autoimmune disease is swelling in the front of the throat, which is known as a goiter. Hashimoto's generally progresses slowly over the course of years, but can cause significant damage to the thyroid.

The Symptoms of
Hashimoto's Thyroiditis

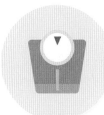

Weight Gain

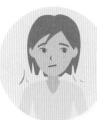

Hair loss or
Little hair

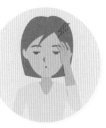

Fatigue

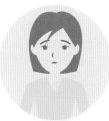

Paleness

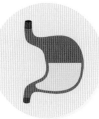

Constipation

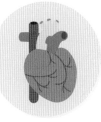

Slowed
heart rate

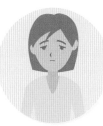

Depression

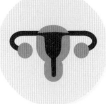

Having a hard
time getting
pregnant

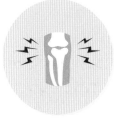

Joint and
muscle pain

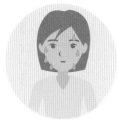

Feeling cold and
having a hard time
getting warm

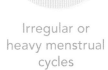

Irregular or
heavy menstrual
cycles

SUBCLINICAL HYPOTHYROIDISM: A condition that is subclinical is a disease that is in the early stages and there may not be any noticeable clinical symptoms. Subclinical hypothyroidism occurs when thyroid-stimulating hormone (TSH) levels are elevated, but thyroid hormone levels are still normal. Elevated TSH normally means that your thyroid is not making enough thyroid hormone, but in the case of subclinical hypothyroidism the TSH is elevated and the thyroid hormones are still in normal ranges. This condition is actually fairly common, and according to an analysis of the National Health and Nutrition Examination Study (NHANES III) data, it can occur in 4.3 percent of the American adult population.

The problem with subclinical hypothyroidism is that there is some controversy surrounding whether or not it indicates a true problem that needs to be treated. There have been some studies that have found that some patients who have been diagnosed with subclinical hypothyroidism have higher cholesterol levels, as well as elevated C-reactive protein. Subclinical hypothyroidism has also been linked to a higher risk of cardiovascular disease. Treating this condition has been shown to help improve certain cardiovascular markers, which is why subclinical hypothyroidism should be examined and taken seriously.

WHY YOUR DOCTOR'S BLOOD TESTS MAY NOT BE UNCOVERING YOUR THYROID CONDITION

How many times have you had your thyroid levels checked, only to be told everything is normal, yet you suffer from all the classic symptoms? You probably wonder why you suffer from chronic fatigue, thinning hair, and even memory issues, but your doctor still claims that everything is exactly where it needs to be regarding your thyroid health. Frustrating, I know!

I can't tell you how many times I have patients come to see me who have all of the symptoms of hypothyroidism but test after test, their doctor tells them that their thyroid levels are within the normal range. Not only is this incredibly frustrating for patients, but the way hypothyroidism is also being tested for can halt the recovery process. When I have patients come to me with all of the classic symptoms who are at their wits' end yet have normal blood tests, I always retest them using a different approach. More often than not, their labs are out of the functional range, and they have positive antibody tests. These antibodies develop when the immune system starts to target the thyroid gland. The test for thyroid antibodies is called the thyroid peroxidase (TPO) antibody test.

The issue with the lab tests used today is that the thyroid ranges are too wide, and physicians are performing incomplete testing. This is the primary reason why people aren't being diagnosed with thyroid issues early on. Most physicians will only test for TSH or TSH and T4 free levels, but in reality, we need a complete thyroid panel to really make an appropriate diagnosis.

In fact, without the proper testing, it's very likely that your thyroid condition will go undetected. Why? Because 95 percent of hypothyroidism is due to Hashimoto's disease, which starts out with inflammation of the thyroid. This condition could take years to develop into hypothyroidism, and early indicators of this condition include high levels of thyroid peroxidase (TPO) and thyroglobulin (Tg) antibodies. But antibody testing is not standard practice.

About 20 percent of patients with Hashimoto's will never have positive antibodies on their labs, but could still have Hashimoto's disease. In fact, in an NHANES study, TPO antibodies were measured, but 20 percent of patients who did have mildly-increased TSH levels did not ever produce thyroid antibodies. This means that this test could be performed over and over again and they would never receive a positive test despite the fact that they still had autoimmune thyroid disease. To confirm the diagnosis in this particular study, a thyroid ultrasound was performed. Skilled practitioners who have experience working with thyroid conditions recognize that in some cases thyroid antibodies may actually never be present on lab tests. This does not always mean that Hashimoto's isn't present. As mentioned, ultrasound can be used to confirm a diagnosis if lab values are negative for thyroid antibodies. Occasionally antibodies are present and a thyroid ultrasound is negative, or antibodies are negative and a thyroid ultrasound is positive. Each patient is unique, so using many different testing mechanisms is important.

The bottom line here is that it's very common that a thyroid condition could go undiagnosed. I have many patients come to me with the classic symptoms but no positive diagnosis. It takes much more than one lab value or one blood test to rule out Hashimoto's. If we only used the clinical findings, it's very possible that doctors would misdiagnose Hashimoto's or completely overlook it more than half of the time.

As I have been mentioning, another big issue with the thyroid tests commonly used today is the fact that the ranges are far too broad. There are two ranges used when looking at blood chemistry: conventional medicine and functional medicine. The conventional medicine range is used to actually diagnose disease, whereas the functional medicine range helps to assess risk for disease as well as uncover these risks before the condition turns into a full-blown disease. When your physician orders lab work, the results are likely interpreted using the conventional medicine range. For example, if your doctor orders a TSH level test, that normal range can vary from 0.5 to 4.5 for most labs. This does not take into account the functional range at all! This only tells you that if you fall within that huge range, then everything is normal, but is it really? The short answer is no. The functional range for TSH as determined by the Endocrine Society is roughly 0.5 to 2.0. You can see the functional range is much more narrow than the conventional range. The Whickham Survey found that there is an increased chance of developing hypothyroidism when TSH is higher than 2.0, which is the upper limit in the functional range. This survey also found that 80 percent of patients who had TSH levels higher than 2.0 produced antibodies. Keep in mind that not everyone with a TSH of 2.0 or more will require treatment. Functional lab ranges are only one of the variables used when it comes to diagnosis; however, it does warrant attention when levels start to go above that range.

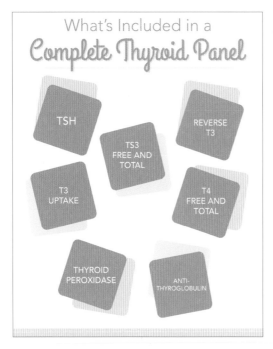

What's Included in a
Complete Thyroid Panel

TSH

REVERSE T3

TS3 FREE AND TOTAL

T3 UPTAKE

T4 FREE AND TOTAL

THYROID PEROXIDASE

ANTI-THYROGLOBULIN

TSH levels are very individualized, and can also vary to some degree. An individual's specific set point may be determined by many different factors. Genetics and environmental factors can play a role in determining what someone's TSH set point may be, and TSH levels may vary with age as well as ethnicity.

Also problematic about physicians only diagnosing thyroid disease based on the conventional medicine range is that it's been noted that there could be an increased risk for cardiovascular disease when TSH values are even slightly elevated. For example, a TSH level of 3 to 4.5 could put you at an increased risk of cardiovascular disease, but using the conventional model would still consider this lab reading to be within the normal range. Having untreated thyroid dysfunction can also pose other health complications, such as kidney dysfunction, psychological issues, heart failure, or worsening diabetes.

Hashimoto's may also go undetected at first glance because TSH levels can fluctuate significantly. This is especially true during the early stages of Hashimoto's because there is commonly a large amount of relapsing and then remission. During an active immune attack, thyroid tissue can be destroyed, leading to a release of some of the thyroid hormones into the bloodstream. This can lead to depressed TSH and even a hyperthyroid state. However, after that period passes, the thyroid would have lost even more of its ability to make thyroid hormone, which would eventually lead to hypothyroidism and TSH levels would go up again. The TSH levels can vary drastically, so it's important to have a practitioner with experience in Hashimoto's and other thyroid conditions. It's not ever as clear as a simple diagnostic blood test to make an appropriate diagnosis.

Lastly, another scenario where diagnosing Hashimoto's can become difficult and may go overlooked is in the case of secondary hypothyroidism. In this case, there are often normal TSH levels but low T4 or T3 levels. In this case, secondary hypothyroidism may be present due to a malfunction of either the hypothalamus or the pituitary gland. This can then lead to a decrease in the activity of the thyroid.

The onset of Hashimoto's is generally seen between the ages of 30 and 50 years old. However, this does not mean that thyroid antibodies cannot show up earlier. If you have had some lab work that may indicate a potential thyroid imbalance or your symptoms are indicative of a thyroid issue, and you have someone in your family with Hashimoto's, it's important to follow that closely. Genes do play a role here, and in fact, if you have a sibling with an autoimmune thyroid disease you are at a higher risk. With studies, it's been shown that nearly 70 percent of Hashimoto's is genetic.

Diagnosing Hashimoto's early is key to getting into remission faster. Early interventions are critical for anyone presenting with thyroid issues. It's important to follow up if you are experiencing any thyroid-related symptoms or seeing imbalances in your lab values that your doctor doesn't necessarily take seriously. Because genetics can play a role, it is critical to work with someone who takes a thorough family history and understands that the risk of thyroid disease can be higher if autoimmune thyroid conditions run in the family.

NEXT STEPS

So, what does this all mean? It means that although your doctor may tell you that your results are "normal," your symptoms are probably telling you otherwise, and your functional range may not be "normal" at all.

Thyroid conditions are also not as easily diagnosed as many doctors portray them to be. It takes some serious detective work and requires working with someone who has extensive experience working with thyroid health. Another common issue I see is that many doctors do not take into account that thyroid receptors are all over the body, and all of our tissues, cells, and organs need functional thyroid hormone levels in order to perform at their best. The thyroid blood tests commonly performed today only measure the level of thyroid hormones present in the blood. Now, remember that all of the cells in our body require thyroid hormone, but these tests do not measure thyroid hormone in the cells or even the amount that your cells are using. As a result, you may have symptoms of hypothyroidism because you may suffer from hypothyroidism at a cellular level, yet have completely normal thyroid ranges according to your blood levels. There are a number of different reasons your thyroid hormones could be blocked from getting into your cells. Some of the common causes include anemia and estrogen dominance, which is why I stress that it's critical to work with someone who has extensive experience in this field to help you get on the road to recovery.

All of these reasons are why so many people end up taking thyroid medications for the rest of their lives. Patients aren't getting diagnosed until there is so much damage to their thyroid that there is no other option but medication. If the proper testing had been done, many patients could have been diagnosed in the early stages, could have gotten control over the condition sooner, and could have been feeling better faster. If you do already have too much damage to your thyroid to produce enough hormones, I cannot stress enough that you must take your medications. However, even if you are on medication, you can benefit by following my 30-Day Thyroid Reset Plan.

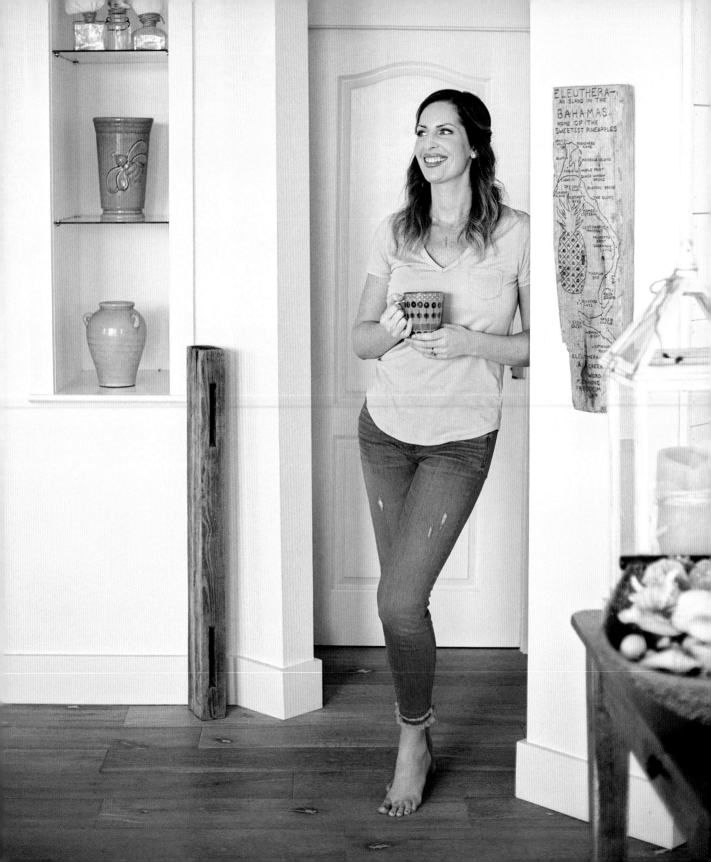

two

UNCOVERING THE SEVEN TRIGGERS THAT ARE KEEPING YOU SICK

If you are experiencing all of the classic symptoms of Hashimoto's, but your blood work consistently comes back normal, then you need to get to the root cause and find what your trigger may be. This is where a functional medicine practitioner comes in. We take the time to examine all the facets of your health. This is incredibly important because if you catch the condition early, there's a chance you may never need to take medication to treat it. With dietary, lifestyle, and supplemental changes, it's very possible to manage this condition before it spirals out of control.

Depending on each patient's situation and what is going on, the treatment plan will vary. We have to remember that treating an autoimmune condition takes a whole-body approach. Even if we are working on the underlying trigger at its source, it's not going to get us the results that we want if we don't address things like sleep and stress. Just keep this in mind as you follow along throughout the rest of the book. A holistic approach is the only way to go about healing from the inside out.

CHRONIC
INFECTIONS

GUT
INFECTIONS

SEX
HORMONE
DYSFUNCTION

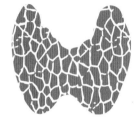

LEAKY GUT
AND FOOD
SENSITIVITIES

Common Triggers of

Hashimoto's

HEAVY METAL
TOXICITY

VITAMIN
DEFICIENCIES

HPA-AXIS
IMBALANCE

When it comes to root causes, there are quite a few, and each person may have one, or they may have multiple triggers. There are seven triggers that may be keeping you sick. These seven triggers include gut infections, leaky gut/food sensitivities, vitamin deficiencies, HPA-axis dysfunction, heavy metal toxicity, sex hormone dysfunction, and chronic infections.

Other Hashimoto's triggers are blood sugar dysregulation, immune dysregulation, environmental toxicities, or reduced oxygen deliverability. Let's dive deeper into the seven most common triggers, and I'll explain how they all relate to the thyroid and Hashimoto's.

TRIGGER 1: GUT INFECTIONS

Believe it or not, your gut has more to do with your health than you may think. In fact, Hippocrates said: "All disease begins in the gut." That was nearly 2,500 years ago, and that saying is still true. The gut, or the gastrointestinal tract, starts at the mouth and ends at the anus. The gut processes food, absorbs nutrients, and houses a large part of the immune system. The gut is so important that more and more research is being conducted on its connection to the brain! Yes, you heard that right: our digestive system may have a lot to do with how we feel mentally, which is why it's no surprise that the gut would have a connection to the thyroid as well. With an imbalanced gut can come an imbalance in many other areas of your health.

Poor gut health leads to thyroid suppression, which can trigger Hashimoto's disease. It's a vicious cycle because low thyroid function can lead to gut inflammation and even leaky gut syndrome. Poor gut health can be in the form of an imbalance in gut bacteria, chronic gut infections, or even leaky gut. First, let's talk about gut bacteria.

Did you know that just one important role of gut bacteria includes assisting in the conversion of inactive T4 into the active form of the thyroid hormone T3? Roughly 20 percent of T4 is converted into T3 in the gastrointestinal tract. In order for this conversion to happen, the gut needs an enzyme called intestinal sulfatase, which comes from healthy gut bacteria. Can you see where the conversion process would run into issues with poor gut bacteria?

With a condition called dysbiosis, there is an imbalance between pathogenic and healthy gut bacteria. Dysbiosis can significantly reduce the conversion of T4 into T3. Here is one of the primary reasons why those who have poor gut health may have very normal lab results but still suffer from classic thyroid symptoms.

Gut Infections

1. Parasites

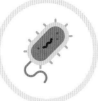

Causes: Contaminated food and water, consuming undercooked meat.

2. Small Intestine Bacterial Overgrowth (SIBO)

Causes: Low stomach acid, long-term proton pump inhibitor use, multiple courses of antibiotics, having diabetes mellitus or Crohn's disease.

3. Yeast

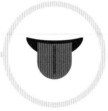

Causes: Corticosteroid use, multiple courses of antibiotics, a high-sugar diet, the birth control pill, chronic stress.

4. Hypochlorhydria

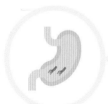

Causes: Overuse of antibiotics, *H. pylori* infection, chronic stress, poor diet, proton pump inhibitors, overuse of nonsteroidal anti-inflammatory drugs, SIBO, food sensitivities.

5. Leaky Gut

Causes: Food sensitivities, gluten consumption, inflammatory foods, candida, intestinal parasites, SIBO, chronic stress, environmental toxins such as mercury and pesticide exposure.

The gut is also home to 70 to 80 percent of immune tissue in the body! Isn't that amazing that more than half of our immune system is in our gut? Here's another reason to take care of your digestive system. The portion of the immune system in the gut is referred to as the gut-associated lymphoid tissue (GALT). This part of the immune system houses many different types of lymphatic tissue that also stores immune cells such as T and B cell lymphocytes. These types of lymphocytes are responsible for producing antibodies against antigens that help the immune system recognize and then go after threats to the body, such as viruses and bacteria.

Gut infections such as small intestinal bacterial overgrowth (SIBO) are another issue. Low stomach acid, also known as hypochlorhydria, can cause SIBO. Atrophic body gastritis, another condition related to low stomach acid, has been linked to Hashimoto's. Other gut infections include yeast overgrowth, bacterial dysbiosis, and parasites. Constipation and inflammation can all impact thyroid function as well.

Suffering from poor gut health can trigger an endless list of health conditions, and thyroid disease is no exception. If you suffer from classic thyroid symptoms, but your doctor has not been able to find that missing link yet, it may be time to dive deeper into how your gut may be impacting the situation.

TRIGGER 2: LEAKY GUT AND FOOD SENSITIVITIES

The gut is designed to help prevent undigested foreign substances from getting into the body. What you ingest will either be digested or will pass through stool. This is a very important function of the gastrointestinal tract, as we do not want undigested foreign substances freely flowing through our body.

Leaky gut occurs when the intestinal barrier fails, or becomes leaky, and allows large protein molecules into the bloodstream. Particles that the gut was supposed to be keeping out are now getting into the body and wreaking havoc on our health. Because the body interprets these large molecules as foreign, the immune system responds by attacking them. These attacks are potentially responsible for causing Hashimoto's.

Leaky gut and food intolerances are also linked to one another. When undigested food particles and other toxins get directly into the bloodstream, the immune system activates a response to these foreign invaders. This is how the food intolerance develops. This is one reason why it's so important to take care of gut health as part of your Hashimoto's healing protocol. It is also important to know that while leaky gut can cause food intolerances, food intolerance can also lead to leaky gut by causing the tight junctions in the gut to open and allow toxins in. This occurs with gluten consumption. Gluten causes the production of zonulin, a chemical that opens up tight junctions in the gut. This is one of the many reasons I recommend all my patients remove gluten from their diet. Consuming gluten can literally cause your gut to be more permeable. Food intolerances can also cause leaky gut by causing SIBO or inflammation in the gut.

Because leaky gut can lead to autoimmune disease such as Hashimoto's, it's critical to address leaky gut at its source. If you can repair the tight junctions, it's likely you can repair whatever damage has been done. Getting to the root cause is the first step in fixing the problem.

Just like gut infections and leaky gut, food intolerances can play a role in the development of Hashimoto's disease as well. Food intolerances are different than food allergies because they do not stimulate an allergic, or immunoglobulin E (IgE), immune reaction. In fact, after ingesting a trigger food, you may not immediately experience any symptoms at all. The reaction may come hours or days later, or not at all if only a small amount was consumed. Symptoms generally develop gradually and can include headaches, diarrhea, bloating, and gas. One cause of a food intolerance is an absence of a specific enzyme that can make digesting a particular food difficult. Food intolerances can also develop due to histamines present in certain foods, such as vinegar.

When it comes to Hashimoto's and food intolerance, it's very possible to have both, and one may mask itself as the other, making it difficult to diagnose. There is also a connection between celiac disease and hypothyroidism, so having one or the other could very well mean you may have both. A study done by Dr. Alessio Fasano found that half of those with celiac disease also had thyroid disease. It's important to get tested for both in this case.

What about a link between food intolerance and Hashimoto's? Can food intolerance lead to an autoimmune thyroid condition? Well, as it turns out with food intolerances, different foods can cause inflammation. The interesting thing is that the IgG branch is the exact same branch that is thought to create thyroid antibodies in numerous cases of Hashimoto's. Consuming foods that cause reactivity and inflammation in the gut can lead to malabsorption of nutrients and leaky gut, which we now know is a trigger of Hashimoto's.

When you identify and then eliminate your intake of reactive foods, you will likely notice a massive improvement in symptoms. People whose thyroid was being impacted may even see a reduction in thyroid antibodies. Amazingly, some people may go into a complete remission once these reactive foods are eliminated! While you cannot get rid of a genetic tendency to autoimmune disorders, remission—the elimination of symptoms—is certainly achievable. Although there may be other triggers, identifying food triggers is a huge step in the right direction and may not only help thyroid function but your overall health as well.

While mainstream medical practices do not often offer these food intolerance tests, functional medicine practitioners can provide these tests, and once the food intolerances are detected, a healing protocol can be started. In my practice, I do not test for food intolerances until we treat the gut, because gut issues can exacerbate food intolerances. It is important to get your gut health in tip-top shape in order to get an accurate read on food intolerance testing. It is also important to keep in mind that not all of these tests are created equal. I have found many of them to be inaccurate. I personally use and have found Cyrex labs to be the most accurate.

TRIGGER 3: VITAMIN DEFICIENCIES

Vitamin deficiencies are another common cause of thyroid disease, yet often go unaccounted for. Vitamin deficiencies can easily go undetected without the proper blood work, and they can easily be mistaken for other conditions.

Vitamin D deficiency has been associated with many different autoimmune diseases, and this particular vitamin plays an important role in thyroid function. Vitamin D helps balance the Th1 (cell-mediated) and Th2 (humoral) parts of the immune system, and it influences T-regulatory cells. Not only that, but a vitamin D deficiency has been specifically associated with autoimmune thyroid disease. A study published by the National Institutes of Health (NIH) determined that vitamin D insufficiency was significantly higher in cases of Hashimoto's thyroiditis than the healthy controls used in the study. While further studies need to be done to determine if vitamin D deficiency is a factor in the development of the disease or if it's just a consequence of Hashimoto's itself, it's very clear that the two are related.

So, you may be thinking, I'll just take some vitamin D, and my issue will be resolved. Unfortunately, for those with thyroid disease, it's not so easy. Because this vitamin is absorbed in the small intestine, those with leaky gut or inflammation in the gastrointestinal tract may not be able to absorb vitamin D properly. For those with thyroid disease, having leaky gut and inflammation in the gut is quite common. Inflammation of any kind also reduces the utilization of vitamin D, as does not eating enough fat or not digesting fat properly.

As you can see, rebalancing vitamin D levels may not be as easy as one would think. When it comes to thyroid conditions, it's important to get other things in check, such as gut health, inflammation, and diet, and then the deficiency can be addressed. This could ultimately boost the health and the function of the thyroid gland if vitamin deficiencies are one of your root causes.

Many people connect thyroid conditions with the need to supplement with iodine, but is that the case? When it comes to the thyroid, iodine deficiency is the most common cause of hypothyroidism worldwide. This was the reason for adding iodine to table salt. However, the outcome wasn't as expected. In fact, in the countries that added iodine to salt, autoimmune thyroid disease increased in prevalence. Why? It turns out that an increase in iodine can actually cause an autoimmune attack on the thyroid. This is especially true for iodine in supplement form. Iodine will actually reduce thyroid peroxidase (TPO), and TPO is needed for thyroid hormone production. However, restricting iodine can reverse hypothyroidism. With that being said, iodine may only cause an issue for those with Hashimoto's or other autoimmune thyroid diseases when they also have a selenium deficiency. Studies have even shown that adequate selenium intake can protect the thyroid from the effects of iodine toxicity. Getting tested for iodine deficiencies, selenium levels, and Hashimoto's may be beneficial, and if an iodine deficiency is present, supplementing with iodine and selenium together may be more beneficial and could potentially help prevent toxicity. Selenium also plays a role in producing thyroid hormone T3.

It's also much better to get selenium from food sources. While selenium supplementation may be key for proper thyroid health, long-term supplementation with high doses of selenium can result in gastrointestinal upset, hair loss, fatigue, irritability, or mild nerve damage. Supplementing with selenium when iodine levels are low can also aggravate hypothyroidism. It's a very delicate balance between these two nutrients. For this reason, the best option is eating a paleo-style diet with lots of selenium-rich foods.

SELENIUM-RICH FOODS

- Brazil nuts—A little goes a long way here; in fact, you only need 1 or 2 per day!
- Sardines
- Halibut
- Grass-fed beef
- Boneless turkey
- Beef liver
- Chicken
- Eggs
- Spinach

A great way to get enough iodine is with a kelp supplement. Remember that selenium and iodine work together, so if using a kelp supplement try to increase your selenium-rich food intake. I will talk much more about both iodine and selenium supplementation in the thyroid supplement section. Be sure to read that section before adding any new supplements to your routine.

TRIGGER 4: HPA-AXIS IMBALANCE

The hypothalamic-pituitary-adrenal (HPA) axis is responsible for helping us adapt to stress. In response to stress, cortisol is released for several hours after encountering the stressor. Cortisol is a hormone that is made by the adrenal glands and is best known for its involvement in the fight-or-flight response. We need cortisol for the body to function properly, but when we are constantly stressed the HPA axis gets desensitized, leading to chronic stress on the hypothalamus, pituitary gland, and adrenal glands.

So, what causes HPA-axis dysfunction? There are many different aspects of our lifestyle that can cause this. Stressors, meaning anything that causes wear and tear on the body, can trigger it. This includes physiological, emotional, physical, and environmental stressors. This also includes stressors that may not make someone feel emotionally or physically stressed, including stressors one may not feel. Things like gut infections and food intolerances all cause the body stress and can cause HPA-axis dysfunction. According to Dr. Guilliams, who wrote the book *The Role of Stress and the HPA Axis in Chronic Disease Management*, there are four categories of stressors that can lead to this HPA-axis dysfunction. Let's take a look at the four categories:

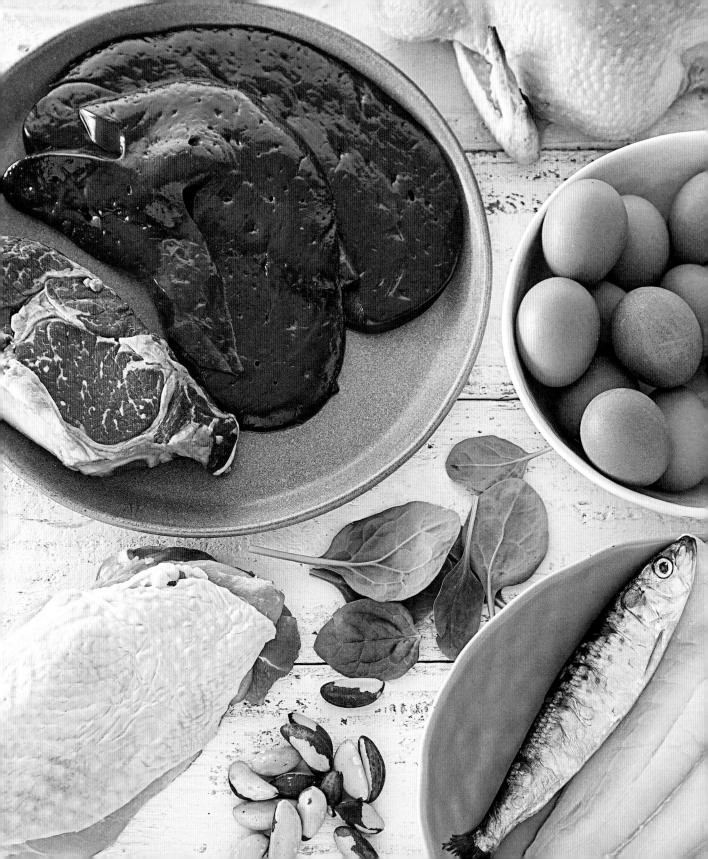

PERCEIVED STRESS

The HPA axis can easily be triggered by signals outside the body that are nonphysical, which the brain perceives as threatening. Public speaking, financial and relationship trouble, or work stress are called "perceived stressors" because how people perceive the event has the ability to affect HPA axis function.

CIRCADIAN DISRUPTION

Circadian rhythms are physical, mental, and behavioral changes that follow a roughly 24-hour cycle, responding primarily to light and darkness in an organism's environment. The HPA axis is intimately tied to the mechanisms controlling circadian rhythm. Unfortunately, most people have the ability to ignore circadian rhythms when choosing their work, social, sleeping, and entertainment schedules. Working the night shift and sleeping during the day, not getting enough sunlight during the day, and the use of electronics at night can lead to HPA-axis dysfunction or other metabolic dysfunctions like obesity and insulin resistance.

GLYCEMIC DYSREGULATION

Glycemic dysregulation is the inability of your body to regulate your blood sugar levels, which can lead to hyper- or hypoglycemia. Poor diet, lack of exercise, and lack of sleep can cause glycemic dysregulation. Cortisol is very important for regulating glucose. When stress happens, the body raises cortisol levels and therefore can increase blood sugar levels. The rising epidemic of insulin resistance, obesity, and related metabolic disorders has a complex cause-and-effect relationship with the increase of stress-related disorders.

INFLAMMATORY SIGNALING

Cortisol is a powerful anti-inflammatory steroid. When someone has chronic inflammation, their body will signal the HPA axis to secrete more cortisol in order to decrease the inflammation. The increase in cortisol downregulates inflammatory pathways within tissues and immune cells through genomic and nongenomic signaling. This suppresses most other immune functions, which explains side effects such as lower resistance to infection. Inflammation from food allergies, obesity, rheumatic diseases, or other factors can be HPA-axis stressors.

It's important to support the HPA axis when it comes to chronic disease management. You must support the central nervous system, the adrenal glands, and how cortisol functions within the tissue. It is especially important for thyroid health because the adrenal glands and the thyroid run on the same axis and both can affect one another. You can begin to do this by removing known stressors and modifying your diet and lifestyle. Working with a functional medicine practitioner can help uncover other potential stressors like food intolerances, heavy metal toxicity, or vitamin deficiency.

TRIGGER 5: HEAVY METAL TOXICITY

This is one of my favorite root causes to talk about because through my experience and the research I have done this is almost always the number one cause of Hashimoto's disease.

Exposure to twenty-three different environmental metals can lead to mercury toxicity. Some of the more common metals include lead, mercury, aluminum, and arsenic, and too much exposure can lead to significant health issues. Toxicity can cause damage to the nervous system as well as organs. The three leading symptoms are chronic fatigue, anxiety, and underactive thyroid—specifically under-conversion of T4 into T3.

Mercury has been of particular interest when it comes to how it affects thyroid health. It's been found that exposure to mercury is linked with cellular autoimmunity as well as the accumulation of mercury within the thyroid gland. A study found that women with mercury exposure had a greater chance of thyroglobulin autoantibody positivity. There have also been studies on the removal of dental amalgams and a reduction in anti-TPO and anti-Tg autoantibodies in those with autoimmune thyroiditis. According to one study, it is very clear that proper removal of dental amalgams in anyone with a mercury hypersensitivity could show significant benefits when it comes to autoimmune thyroid disease. It's also very clear that there is a real connection between mercury exposure and overall thyroid health.

Some common risk factors for heavy metal toxicity include living in a home with lead-based paint, consuming fish high in mercury, inhaling tobacco smoke, or having dental amalgam fillings. If you are exposed to more than one of these things, your risk goes up even higher.

Consuming fish is a very common way people are exposed to mercury. Because mercury has been linked to cellular autoimmunity, it's really important to keep mercury exposure to a minimum. When choosing which fish to add into your diet, steer away from high-mercury options like ahi tuna, orange roughy, shark, and swordfish, among others.

If you are suffering from heavy metal toxicity, it's crucial that you get treated as soon as possible, as untreated toxicities can lead to chronic health conditions, such as chronic fatigue syndrome and fibromyalgia. A functional medicine practitioner can get you on the right path with testing and treatment options. Some common testing options include blood tests, urinalysis testing, and hair and nail analysis.

TRIGGER 6: SEX HORMONE DYSFUNCTION

Sex hormone dysfunction is another common underlying trigger of Hashimoto's thyroiditis. Hashimoto's disease does affect more women than men, and many people who suffer from Hashimoto's also have something called estrogen dominance. This is actually an imbalance between estrogen and progesterone. This can be caused by an excess of estrogen, but more likely it's caused by too little progesterone. Estrogen dominance can either directly cause or contribute to a thyroid or an autoimmune thyroid condition. Many women who have estrogen dominance may very well have accompanying thyroid issues. Estrogen can affect the conversion of T4 into T3, which could ultimately result in low T3 levels. Symptoms of hypothyroidism can occur due to an estrogen dominance in this case. Hypothyroid symptoms can also arise when estrogen dominance blocks the uptake of thyroid hormone. T4 and T3 levels can also be very low because, in the presence of estrogen dominance, thyroid-binding globulin can become increased. This is the protein that helps carry thyroid hormones to the cells. T3 and T4 get attached to thyroid-binding globulin, resulting in T3 and T4 levels being low.

Unfortunately, estrogen dominance suppresses the immune system and can lead to the development of Hashimoto's disease. Women who are experiencing perimenopause or going through menopause need to pay particular attention to progesterone levels during this time because they tend to plummet while estrogen levels stay the same. This can cause estrogen dominance and ultimately a thyroid condition. It's critical to get these hormones tested to determine whether a sex hormone imbalance is causing the thyroid condition, and then work to get them back in balance.

A functional medicine practitioner can help with getting the hormones back in balance by addressing lifestyle and dietary changes. Because chronic stress can trigger hormonal imbalance, it's important to implement a stress reduction protocol, avoid environmental toxins, and start a dietary protocol specifically known to balance hormones and nourish the stress response within the body.

All of this is within reach; it's all about starting the proper protocol and catching the issue before it spirals into numerous other problems, because sex hormone dysfunction can cause more than just Hashimoto's disease if left untreated.

TRIGGER 7: CHRONIC INFECTIONS

Chronic infections like Lyme disease, gut infections, hepatitis C, and Epstein-Barr virus can trigger Hashimoto's and other autoimmune conditions. Often many of these chronic infections go undetected by modern physicians because the proper testing may not have been offered, or in many cases, these conditions may appear to be similar to another type of diagnosis. Epstein-Barr virus can be difficult to diagnose because the virus can be dormant in your body and not cause any symptoms. Lyme disease can also be difficult to diagnose because the symptoms associated with Lyme are often nonspecific and may mimic other conditions. Either way, it can make diagnosing these conditions difficult and the longer they are left untreated, the higher your risk for developing something like Hashimoto's.

Keep in mind that while there may not be a cure for some of these infections, there are functional medicine treatment options that can keep the infection at bay. For example, with Epstein-Barr virus it is very important to optimize your sleep; enjoy a diet that includes lots of healing foods such as coconut oil, parsley, cilantro, curcumin, and sweet potatoes; and reduce as much stress as possible. This goes for all chronic infections.

Chronic infections can cause an autoimmune reaction through molecular mimicry. The infection may look like your own body tissue, and when this happens, your immune system starts attacking healthy tissue, including the thyroid. While the infection is active, the immune system will just keep attacking. This is why chronic infections are one of the common triggers of autoimmune conditions such as Hashimoto's thyroiditis and why it's so important to get these infections diagnosed properly. Early intervention is key.

Viruses like Epstein-Barr can lay dormant in your body and then reactivate. When the virus is reactivated, it could cause the production of thyroid antibodies and then lead to further autoimmune symptoms. Another major issue with Epstein-Barr virus is that there are different stages and once stage three starts, the virus begins to settle in the liver and the spleen, and there is a potential for it to settle in other organs of the body, such as the thyroid, as well. The virus could lay dormant in your organs for a number of years, going undetected, which could cause significant inflammation. At this stage, it's very easy for the virus to go undetected and for doctors to overlook that Epstein-Barr virus is even present in the body. It's very likely that blood tests would not show the virus to be active in the bloodstream at this stage. Meanwhile, it could be causing inflammation in various organs in the body.

So, how can Epstein-Barr virus affect the thyroid? Once this virus is in your thyroid, it can start to affect the thyroid tissue. The virus can kill off thyroid cells and can lead to hypothyroidism. When your immune system takes notice of what is going on in the thyroid, it will likely trigger an inflammatory response. Unfortunately, due to the fact that this particular virus is very good at hiding in organs and can release toxins in the body that can cause confusion within the immune system, it can be difficult for the immune system to rid the thyroid of the hidden Epstein-Barr virus.

While it's scary to think that a chronic infection such as Epstein-Barr can have such a significant impact on the health of your thyroid, the thyroid has the amazing ability to heal itself. If chronic infections are one of your triggers, then working with a functional medicine practitioner to help uncover a chronic infection that may be lying dormant in your body is one of the first steps to recovery.

With any chronic infection, it's necessary to treat the infection at its source, not only to help prevent autoimmunity in the first place but also to help reduce the chances of the infection worsening your symptoms.

QUIZ: ARE YOUR CORTISOL LEVELS TOO HIGH?

As a way to wrap up the seven hidden triggers section of this book, I encourage you to take this short quiz. This is a great way to help you determine whether your cortisol levels are high. If they are high, there's a good chance you are suffering from a handful of unwanted symptoms, and not getting cortisol levels back in balance can ultimately lead to adrenal burnout.

As you learned about with trigger number four, HPA-axis imbalance, it's essential to balance cortisol levels when managing any chronic disease.

Find out if Your

Cortisol Levels

are High Quiz

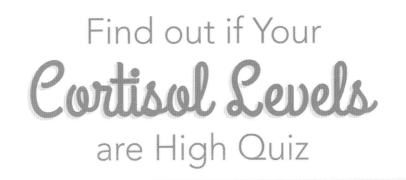

To get started, answer the following questions using the scale:

0 - never   **1 - rarely**   **2 - often**   **3 - almost always**

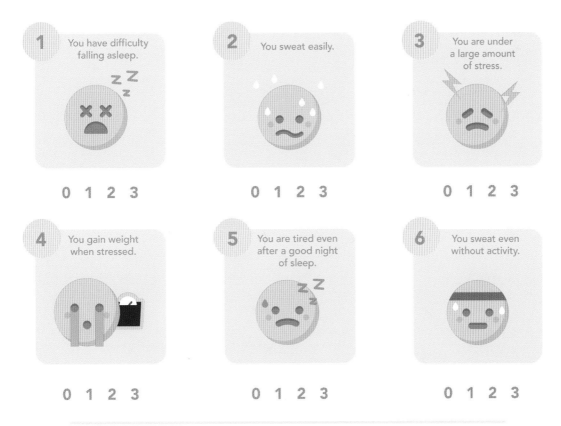

1 You have difficulty falling asleep.

0 1 2 3

2 You sweat easily.

0 1 2 3

3 You are under a large amount of stress.

0 1 2 3

4 You gain weight when stressed.

0 1 2 3

5 You are tired even after a good night of sleep.

0 1 2 3

6 You sweat even without activity.

0 1 2 3

To get your results, follow this guide:

If you picked mostly 0 and 1, then you most likely do not have high cortisol levels.

If you picked mostly 1 and 2, then you may be at risk for having high cortisol levels.

If you picked mostly 2 and 3, then there is a good chance that you have high cortisol levels.

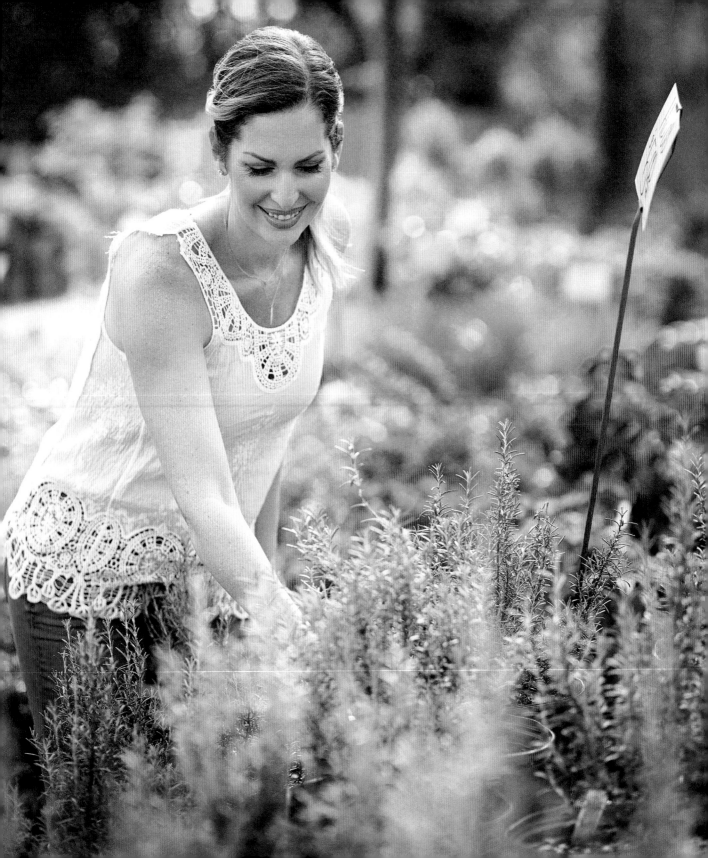

three

GETTING INTO
REMISSION

Getting into remission takes a multifaceted approach. Remission is not the same as a "cure" for Hashimoto's, but remission is when you have uncovered your trigger or triggers, have boosted gut health, and have supported your adrenal glands in order to boost thyroid health. Remission means that you are virtually asymptomatic. Reaching remission does require a holistic approach. For example, just doing one of the recommendations in this section is not likely to make you better. It will certainly help you toward recovery, but one change is not enough to make a long-lasting impact. I have many clients come to my office who have already made changes to their diet by giving up gluten, and they don't notice any difference in the way they feel. While giving up gluten is an integral part of the healing process, it's only one piece to a very complicated puzzle. This is not meant to discourage you, but I do want you to know that there are many steps involved in getting well and all of them are very attainable—you just have to know how to implement them!

GETTING THE PROPER TESTING

One of the very first steps to getting into remission is getting the proper testing. Even if you've had thyroid tests done through your primary medical doctor, thyroid conditions can still be present with normal blood values. Much depends on the type of test you get done. Different tests can check for various things. For example, you can tell a lot by performing a urinalysis for a heavy metal toxicity or checking the blood for food sensitivities. Many tests are very specific and something that functional medicine practitioners can offer for individual needs. Here are just a handful of tests that can be conducted to help get to your root cause:

- Heavy metal testing
- Food sensitivity and allergy testing
- Hormone testing
- Dried urine testing
- Thyroid level check

- Methylation testing
- Immunological testing
- Stool testing
- Leaky gut testing
- SIBO breath testing

With proper testing, you can get to the bottom of what's truly going on and start on a path of healing. The great thing about these tests is that they allow for an individualized approach. Whatever the lab results show will help guide you in creating a healing protocol that will work best for you.

With that being said, let's jump right in and talk about some of the other important steps in starting your own Hashimoto's recovery process.

REMOVING TOXINS FROM YOUR EVERYDAY LIFE

Our bodies are so inundated with toxins on a daily basis that we must reduce the total toxin burden to begin the healing process. Constant exposure to irritants prevents the immune system from doing what it is supposed to do. Instead, it remains in a hyperactive state trying to fight off everything around it, including healthy tissue. In addition to stress on the immune system, many toxins are endocrine disrupters. An endocrine disrupter is a hormone-altering chemical that can either increase or decrease the production of certain hormones in the body. Endocrine disruptors can also mimic other hormones, which can lead to hormonal imbalances. These disruptors can also build up in body organs, which is why it is so important to remove them from your everyday life.

Making your environment cleaner is a balancing act, and it all takes time. For now, focus on taking baby steps toward change.

CIGARETTE SMOKE: Whether you smoke yourself or are exposed to secondhand smoke, this is something that will need to be completely avoided when you start your healing protocol. Smoking can actually trigger certain autoimmune diseases, which is why it's so important to quit smoking if you smoke, and avoid anyone around you who smokes if you suffer from an autoimmune condition.

XENOESTROGENS AND ENVIRONMENTAL ESTROGENS: Environmental estrogens are compounds that mimic estrogen and are abundantly found in the environment. Conventional products from animals treated with hormones and antibiotics will likely contain significant amounts of estrogens. Xenoestrogens are synthetic estrogens that are commonly found in plastics, pesticides, and detergent. Estrogens in very large amounts are harmful to the immune system and can cause endocrine disruption. Limit your exposure by choosing grass-fed and pasture-raised animal products, avoiding dairy, eliminating soy, and choosing glass water bottles and food storage containers over plastic containers. You can also switch to all-natural laundry detergents made from plant-based ingredients.

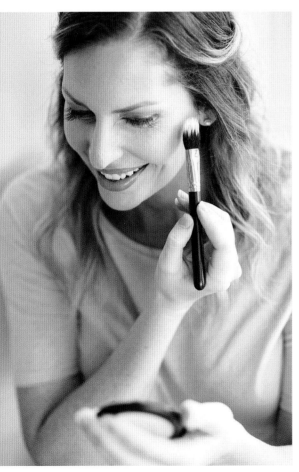

PERSONAL CARE PRODUCTS: Many personal care products contain endocrine disruptors. While we would hope that the moisturizer we put on our skin or the deodorant we use would be safe, this isn't always the case. Here are some of the ingredients to watch out for and avoid when choosing a personal care product:

- BISPHENOL-A (BPA)
- PHTHALATES
- PARABENS
- FORMALDEHYDE
- FRAGRANCE/PERFUME
- OXYBENZONE
- DIETHYLENE GLYCOL (DEG)

The best way to avoid these chemicals is to opt for organic, plant-based care products. Many companies are now jumping on the clean bandwagon, but you still should check the ingredient list. Skin care products tend to be the worst culprits, so a great skin care alternative would be witch hazel for cleansing and coconut oil for moisturizing. Makeup products also contain many items on this list. Check the ingredient list carefully before you buy any new product to keep these chemicals out of your body!

HOUSEHOLD CLEANING PRODUCTS: Many of the products sitting under your sink right now may be triggering endocrine disruption. That's because many store-bought products contain chemicals such as:

* Phthalates
* Perchloroethylene (PERC)
* Triclosan
* Fragrance
* Sodium lauryl/laureth sulfate

All of these chemicals can cause significant hormone disruption. The best way to avoid these is to either make your own homemade cleaning products or to check the Environmental Working Group website to see which products are safest to use.

BOTTLED WATER: While many companies are now offering BPA-free water bottles, it still doesn't prevent other chemicals from seeping into the water when the bottle is exposed to heat. Some of the chemicals used in plastic water bottles are known endocrine disruptors, including BBP (benzyl butyl phthalate) and dioxin, which has a strong link to cancer and can interfere with hormones. Stop drinking bottled water and invest in a great at-home water filtration system. If your budget allows, you can get one installed in your home. Otherwise, there are on-the-counter options that are convenient and cost-effective. Berkey water filters are great and last many, many years. Drinking clean water is essential, especially for those with autoimmune disease or other illnesses.

DO-IT-YOURSELF TOXIN-FREE LIVING

Here are some DIY toxin-free recipes to help you avoid common toxins you may be in contact with on a daily basis.

DIY ALL-PURPOSE CLEANER

MAKES 2 CUPS (480 ML)

WHAT YOU NEED

2 cups (480 ml) distilled water

2 tbsp (30 ml) castile soap

15 drops lavender essential oil

Start by pouring the water into a spray bottle (a glass spray bottle is best) followed by the soap and then the essential oil.

Shake and then store as you would traditional cleaner.

Use in place of toxic household cleaners.

DIY HAND SOAP

MAKES 1 CUP (240 ML)

WHAT YOU NEED

½ cup (120 ml) distilled water

½ cup (120 ml) castile soap

1 tbsp (15 ml) olive oil

10 drops peppermint essential oil

Start by adding the water to a hand soap bottle followed by the castile soap.

Add the olive oil and essential oil and gently shake.

Use as a clean-living hand soap.

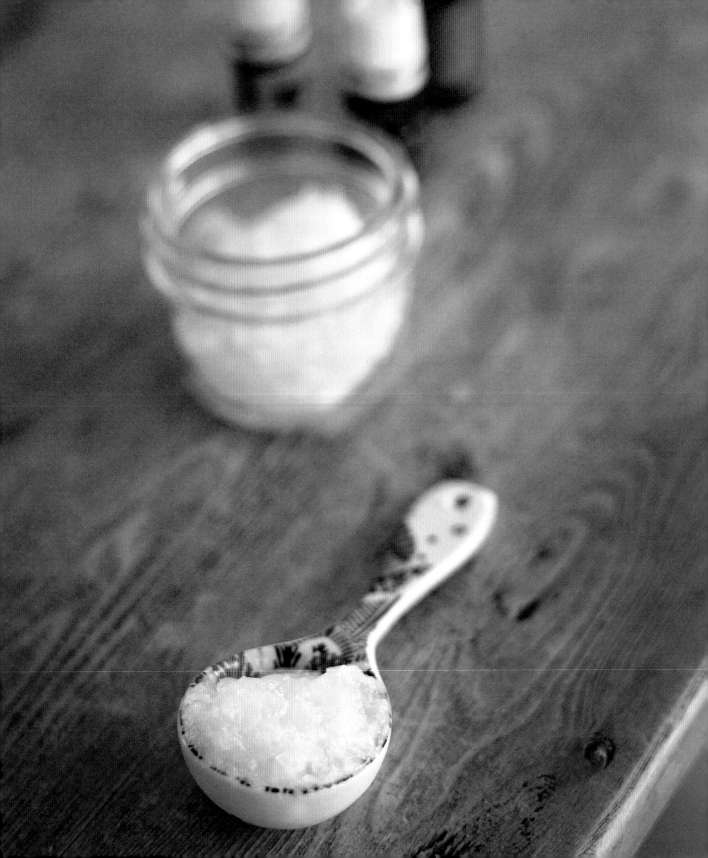

HOMEMADE DEODORANT

MAKES ½ CUP (120 G)

WHAT YOU NEED

¼ cup (60 ml) coconut oil

¼ cup (55 g) baking soda

2 tbsp (16 g) arrowroot flour

10 drops lavender essential oil

Simply mix all the ingredients together in a mixing bowl and store in a glass jar.

Use a nickel-size amount and apply as you would regular deodorant.

If you aren't quite ready to jump into all DIY products, here are some great brands that offer natural alternatives to the traditional chemical-filled products. You can also check out the Environmental Working Group at EWG.org to search personal care or cleaning products and check to see how safe it really is.

- Dr. Bronner's castile soap
- AspenClean all-purpose cleaner
- Attitude all-purpose eco cleaner
- Young Living Thieves household cleaner, dish soap, and laundry detergent
- Better Life laundry detergent, lavender and grapefruit
- Seventh Generation natural laundry detergent powder, free and clear
- Crystal body deodorant
- PurelyGreat cream deodorant
- Beautycounter skin care, makeup, and hair care

YOUR ESSENTIAL OIL GUIDE

I like to talk about essential oils when addressing toxicity because these oils can serve as a great replacement for common chemical-based fragrances.

Whether you currently use essential oils or have been interested in incorporating them into your healing protocol, I strongly advocate their use, especially when they are applied properly and the right types of oils are selected. It is so important to invest in quality and pure essential oils. I personally use and recommend the brand Young Living, because their oils are extremely high quality and they offer some incredible essential oil blends.

Essential oils can enhance both emotional and physical wellness. Many of the blends Young Living offers can help your body restore balance when used in conjunction with a healthy lifestyle and a clean diet. I personally love to use Endoflex by Young Living. I mix this essential oil blend with coconut oil and use it as a lotion. Not only does it smell amazing, but it also helps support the endocrine system. When you use essential oils in place of synthetic chemical products, you help support overall health while also enjoying a beautiful and refreshing fragrance from pure botanicals.

A great blend for thyroid health is 5 drops of lemongrass and 5 drops of clove oil mixed with 3 drops of frankincense oil in about ¼ cup (60 g) of coconut oil and then apply it to the thyroid. Lemongrass mixed with myrrh oil is another great combination for thyroid health. You can start with 2 drops of each mixed with about 1½ tablespoons (23 g) of coconut oil.

Joint pain can be an issue for anyone with Hashimoto's or hypothyroidism, and amazingly, essential oils can help with this ailment as well. Instead of using toxic over-the-counter pain-relieving gels, try investing in a quality essential oil that can directly target joint and muscle pain. Lemongrass and marjoram essential oils mixed with an organic, nontoxic, unscented lotion can make an excellent all-natural pain-relieving gel. Try mixing 15 drops of lemongrass essential oil with 15 drops of marjoram in a bottle of lotion. Use on sore muscles and joints when needed. The key here is to stick to a nontoxic lotion that contains zero fragrance and is paraben-free.

Your Essential Oil Guide

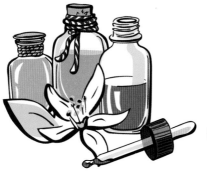

Essential Oils for Fatigue

Rosemary   Eucalyptus
Lemon   Grapefruit
Peppermint   Other citrus scents

Essential Oils for Anxiety & Irritability

Lavender
Chamomile
Frankincense

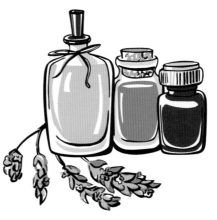

Essential Oils for Hypothyroidism

Frankincense
Lemongrass
Clove

Essential Oils for Joint Pain

Lemongrass
Marjoram

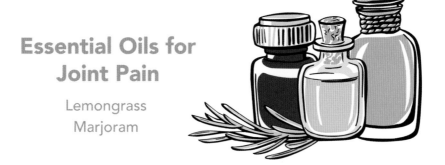

Stress triggers inflammation, can weaken the immune system, and may worsen your symptoms. Therefore, reducing your stress is an important part of treating an autoimmune condition.

When you deal with chronic stress, your body releases cortisol. High levels of cortisol can actually cause the thyroid to have to work harder just to create adequate amounts of thyroid hormone. If your thyroid function is already compromised from an underlying thyroid condition, stress can put an even greater strain on your thyroid, ultimately causing both your thyroid condition and your symptoms to worsen. A study published in the journal *Thyroid* linked stress as one of the environmental factors for thyroid autoimmunity. High levels of stress put your body at a greater risk of developing Hashimoto's.

Below are some of my favorite ways to control stress and restore thyroid health. While some of the items on the list may not seem to be stress management, things like a healthy diet go hand in hand with helping reduce the stress load on your body. If you can treat your body holistically and take care of every aspect of your health, both the physical and the mental burden will be reduced and you will be able to better deal with the stressors we all face in life. Although stress is an inevitable part of life, it's all about how we manage it.

TIPS TO MANAGE YOUR STRESS

Try these methods of managing stress until you find what works best for you.

BE AWARE: Just being aware of your stress levels can have a positive impact on your health. If you go about your day-to-day life not acknowledging the levels of stress you face, the stress will never be addressed. The first step to getting it under control is to determine which areas of your life cause the most stress. If it's your job, you may want to think about ways you can reduce the burden when it comes to work. Maybe you have a really long commute and get stuck in rush hour traffic every morning and on your drive home. While this is not something you may necessarily have too much control over, maybe you can listen to a relaxing podcast during the drive to reduce the stress just a bit. Bringing awareness to the stress levels is the first step here.

BE AWARE OF YOUR BREATH: It is important to be aware of our breath. Many of us hold our breath when we are stressed and uptight. Unfortunately, holding our breath only worsens that tense and anxious feeling. It's only when we are present with the way we breathe and actively work to breathe deeply does stress start to reduce. Try to be present with how you are breathing throughout the day. If you find you are stressed out, take a second to see if you are holding your breath or breathing shallowly. If you are, take four deep breaths in and out and see how that makes you feel. Chances are it will help you center yourself so you can carry on with your day a little less stressed out.

How to Practice
Mindfulness

The first step in the practice of mindfulness is to set some time aside to simply observe the present moment. Just pay attention to what is going on around you. This doesn't mean you have to reach a sense of calm or put judgment on what is going on, just be present with the moment.

Next, let go of any judgments that may come up. If any come up, simply note them and move on instead of letting your mind get stuck on that thought. The point is to just keep returning to the present moment.

Don't be hard on yourself! If you find your mind wandering when you are trying hard to be present, just acknowledge that your mind is wandering to other thoughts and try to re-center yourself to the present moment

That's it! Mindfulness training appears to be simple, and it is after some practice. Give it a try throughout the day, and you may be surprised at the calming effect it can have on your body.

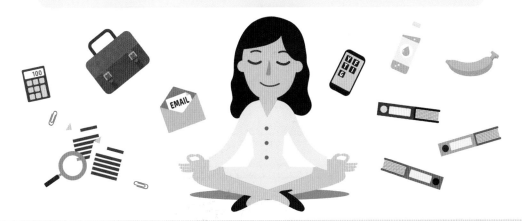

MINDFULNESS TRAINING: Being mindful is about being fully aware of where you are, what you are doing, and not overreacting or being overwhelmed by what is going on around you. While we all have the power to practice mindfulness, practicing it daily makes it that much easier, and it will soon become second nature. Amazingly, training your brain to be more mindful may actually help to remodel the structure of your brain! Think back to the HPA axis section where we talked about perceived stress. So many of us run our lives on autopilot, and our bodies are constantly in that fight-or-flight state even when real threat is not present. The body begins to respond to perceived stress the same way it would respond to serious danger. This can throw your entire body out of whack, including your thyroid. Mindfulness can significantly help here, and the great thing about it is that anyone can do it. It doesn't matter how old you are or if you have any physical limitations.

EAT A HEALTHY DIET: A healthy diet is the foundation of health. Only we are in charge of the food choices we make, and diet plays such an important role in thyroid health. When you consume nourishing and healing foods, it takes unnecessary stress off the body. However, when you consume a diet full of processed and artificial foods, you tax your body even further. Consuming a healthy diet will help your body deal with both emotional and physical stressors.

EXERCISE: Exercise is an important part of a healthy lifestyle, but don't think you have to do anything extreme! Walking, yoga, cycling, jogging—they all count as great ways to get your body moving. You don't need to spend hours in the gym; in fact, when dealing with an autoimmune disease it's best not to overexert yourself. The point is to move your body enough to reduce your stress levels and give yourself a natural boost of energy. Do what feels good and stay consistent with it.

YOGA AND MEDITATION: These are two of the most talked about stress-reducing techniques, because yoga and meditation both have proven health benefits. They are also free and can be practiced anywhere by anybody. Try adding a ten-minute guided meditation and a ten-minute morning yoga sequence to your day to help get your stress levels under control. Eventually, you will build yourself up to do an hour yoga routine and a half hour of meditation. Just start small, and your body will guide you when you are ready to advance to the next level. As a rule of thumb, try to get at least 30 minutes of physical activity each day. Yoga is a low-impact form of exercise, and working your way up to an hour yoga class is a great goal. However, always listen to your body, and if you are only able to work up to 30 minutes at a time, that is totally fine!

Reducing your stress is one of the best ways to help control Hashimoto's. Unfortunately, there is no one single thing you can do that will get you into remission. It takes a multidisciplinary approach involving both the mind and the body, and reducing your stress levels is certainly part of that equation.

TIPS FOR HEALTHY EXERCISE

We all know that exercise is healthy and that incorporating some type of movement into our day-to-day life will help us stay in the best shape possible. However, when you have Hashimoto's or another autoimmune condition, it's important to talk about the type of exercise you should be doing as well as how much. The last thing you want is to burn out your body even more thinking you are doing something healthy, but ultimately having it cause more harm than good.

I recommend taking a two-phase approach with exercise when dealing with Hashimoto's. The first phase involves lighter types of activity, such as yoga, Pilates, and walking. In the first phase, when you are still really symptomatic, the whole point is to just get your body moving and out of a sedentary position. Exercise can help reduce stress, balance blood pressure, ease anxiety, and increase bone density. One of the best ways to get some low-intensity exercise into your day is by walking. You don't even need to walk fast; you just need to walk.

When you are working to get your symptoms under control, too much exercise can be just as bad as not moving your body at all. Too much exercise can cause inflammation and tax the immune system. Some symptoms, such as heart palpitations, shortness of breath, and fatigue, can make it almost impossible to exercise to begin with, so strenuous exercise should really be out of the picture when you are working to get your symptoms under control. It's important to exercise in a way that will boost your energy instead of stripping your body of more.

The second phase of exercise can come after you are feeling good and have supported your thyroid and adrenal glands. Once you feel up to it, including some high-intensity interval training (HIIT) as well as Tabata and CrossFit is okay. All of these exercises can be modified to what you feel you can handle. Keep in mind that when I talk about HIIT and CrossFit, I am not talking about exercise such as marathon training that requires hours of activity at one time. The HIIT I am talking about involves short bursts of activity with rests in between. The high-intensity exercise that you want to avoid are things that require you to train for long periods of time. They can actually cause the body's stress response to go too far, which can lead to biochemical changes that cause damage to overall health for not just the short term but the long term as well. Overtraining can also affect blood levels of 5-HTP, glutamine, and dopamine, which can all lead to increased fatigue, and can affect the hypothalamic-pituitary axis, which can ultimately lead to hypothyroidism. So, when you are feeling up to doing a little higher intensity exercise, try CrossFit (modified if necessary), Tabata, and HIIT, as all of these allow you to rest in between periods of activity. However, if you feel depleted and fatigued after exercising, it means that your body is not quite ready, and you should return to phase one that includes lighter exercises such as walking, yoga, and Pilates.

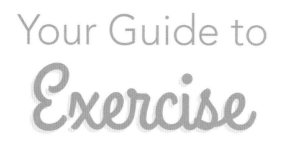

Your Guide to Exercise

Here are some healthy ways to include exercise in your day:

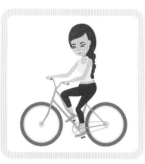

A brisk daily walk

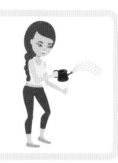

Gardening

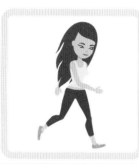

Gentle cycling

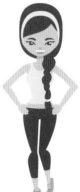

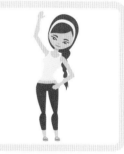

Daily stretching

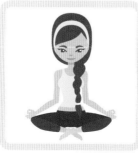

A morning or evening
yoga routine

TIPS FOR RESTFUL SLEEP

Did you know that not getting enough sleep can be a recipe for disaster and can increase stress on the body? A lack of sleep can lead to food cravings, obesity, diabetes, and depression. Getting into bed too late can also lead to poor sleep habits. When you get to bed later than 10:00 or 10:30 at night you run the risk of rising cortisol levels, which can make it very difficult to fall asleep. Typically, when you have balanced cortisol levels, your levels begin to drop in the evening preparing for bed. However, after the 10:00 hour your adrenals may kick into high gear again, giving you a cortisol boost. To prevent this and to promote a restful night's sleep, it is important to set a strict sleep schedule and get to bed early.

Sleep is incredibly important. Sleep helps maintain and repair the nervous, immune, and digestive systems. When you don't get enough sleep, you are more likely to get sick. When you do get a good night's sleep, you improve your immune function, concentration, and stress intolerance, and you will likely have more energy.

When dealing with an autoimmune condition, not getting enough sleep can further stress the immune system, making you even more susceptible to disease. A lack of sleep can lead to low-grade chronic inflammation, and inflammation is at the root of nearly all chronic disease. A study done at UCLA found that even small amounts of sleep loss can trigger both cellular and genetic processes that are involved in the body's inflammatory response to disease. They noted that sleep loss for just one night increased inflammation.

There are many things you can do to try to improve the quality of your sleep, but everyone is unique, so you may need to practice a few of these tips before you find the one or the combination that works best for you.

Your Guide to
Sleep

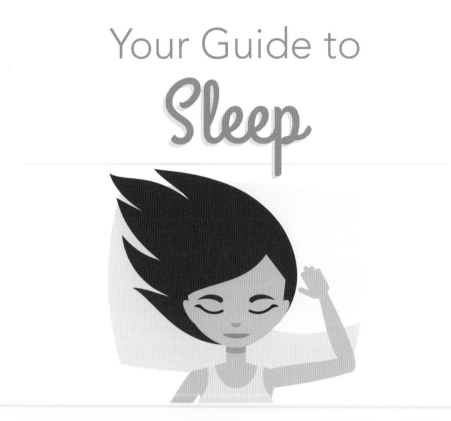

Stay Away from Artificial Light as Much as Possible

Artificial light can throw circadian rhythms out of whack, which in turn disrupts the sleep cycle. To avoid artificial light, strive to stay away from your computer, phone, tablet, and television at least two to three hours before you go to bed. Make your room extra dark with blackout blinds if necessary.

Get into Bed Earlier

The trick here is to get to bed before your cortisol levels spike and keep you awake until all hours of the night. Try to get to bed before 10 p.m.

Make Sure You Ate Enough

No one sleeps well with a growling belly, so it's important to be sure that you ate enough during the day, but also keep in mind that you don't want to go to bed immediately after a meal. If you tend to suffer from hypoglycemia (low blood sugar), you may want to have a high-protein snack, such as a handful of nuts or seeds, an hour before bed to keep your blood sugar levels stable. However, if you suffer from digestive issues, such as acid reflux, try to eat at least two to three hours before bedtime.

Relax

If you feel tense at the end of the day, and your mind spins thinking about all of the things you need to accomplish the next day, you may need to do some relaxation exercises before bed. Try taking a bath or doing a gentle yoga sequence to calm the mind. Do what feels good to wind down the day. For some, it just means sipping on some herbal tea and doing a few minutes of meditation; for others, a solid hour of relaxation may be needed to calm the mind.

DAILY LIFESTYLE AND SELF-CARE TIPS

Here's a handy list for making sure you are meeting all your self-care goals. Make sure you:

- Practice daily stress reduction. Try yoga, meditation, reading, walking, and whatever else helps you reduce stress.
- Practice mindfulness training.
- Swap toxic beauty products for clean options.
- Eliminate toxic cleaning products and make your own or buy green options.
- Get at least eight hours of uninterrupted sleep per night.
- Find joy and do something that makes you happy every day.
- Be social, daily.
- Disconnect at least a few hours before bed by turning off the TV, getting away from the computer, and staying off your phone as much as possible.
- Limit caffeine and opt for herbal teas instead.
- Find time each weekend to take a day to just RELAX!
- Eat bone broth daily.
- Find a support group.
- Get some gentle exercise daily.
- Follow a healthy paleo-style diet.
- Drink enough clean, filtered water each day.
- Show yourself some love each day.
- Organize your daily schedule and eliminate any unnecessary commitments.

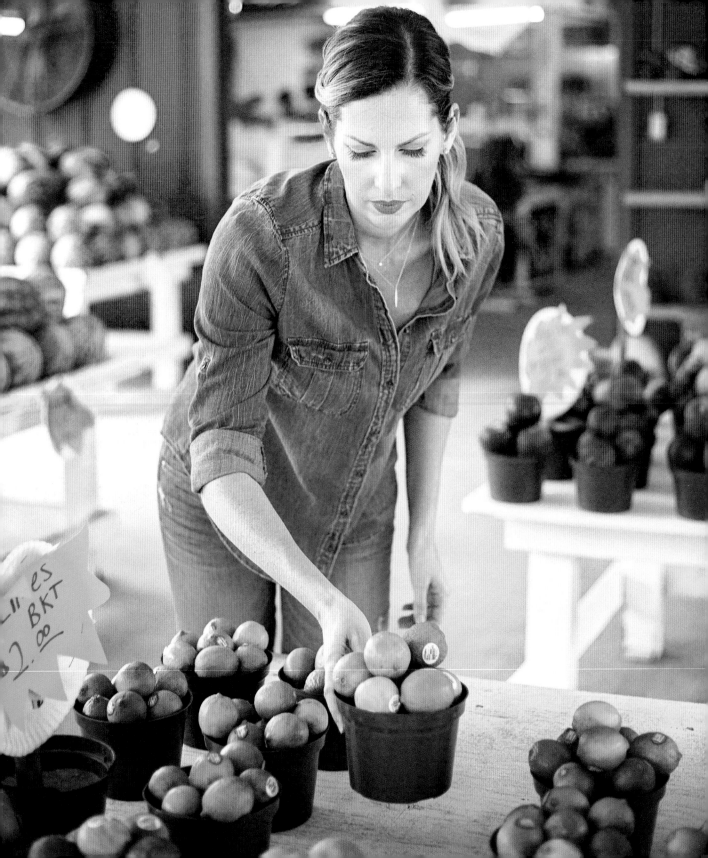

four

THE IMPORTANCE
OF DIET

Diet is an incredibly important part of living a healthy life and is even more important when you are dealing with an autoimmune condition. What you feed your body daily is either going to fuel the disease further or help you toward remission. There are some foods you know your body will not tolerate, and each person is different. However, there are also foods that nearly all people with Hashimoto's disease should steer clear of.

When I consult with clients, I strive to work with them so that they are following the least restrictive diet possible while still consuming foods that support thyroid health and staying away from the foods that detract from thyroid health. Ultimately, each person is different, and everyone will have different dietary requirements. It's important to know that the 30-Day Thyroid Reset is a great starting point, but a paleo-style approach is a realistic long-term dietary goal for anyone with an autoimmune condition. I like to point out that the type of diet I recommend is a paleo-like diet because there are different variations of this diet and some of the foods on the paleo diet aren't going to necessarily work for someone with a thyroid condition. Later in this chapter I will talk about the thyroid reset and why this is a great way to kick-start the healing process. But first, here are some general food categories you should be eating for thyroid health.

Foods for
Thyroid Health

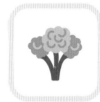

**Organic
vegetables**

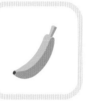

**Green
plantains**

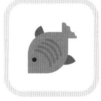

**Wild-caught
fish**

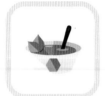

**Bone
broth**

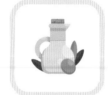

**Coconut
oil**

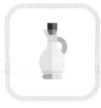

**Olive
oil**

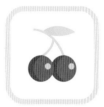

**Low-sugar fruits:
berries, cantaloupe,
cherries**

**Fermented foods:
sauerkraut, kimchi,
unsweetened coconut yogurt,
water kefir**

**Grass-fed and
pasture-raised animal
products**

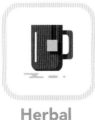

**Herbal
teas**

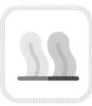

Seaweeds

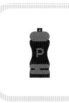

**Herbs and
spices**

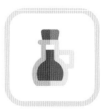

**Apple cider
vinegar**

WHEN TO EAT ORGANIC VERSUS CONVENTIONAL

There are many lists to help you determine which foods contain the largest amount of pesticides and herbicides. While I always recommend you purchase organic whenever possible, that may not always be feasible. Organic produce can be quite pricey and sometimes difficult to find. If that is the case, I recommend that all of my patients follow the Environmental Working Group's Clean Fifteen and Dirty Dozen lists to know which foods they should always purchase organic and which foods may be OK to buy conventional every now and then.

I have included the most current 2017 Clean Fifteen and Dirty Dozen list from the Environmental Working Group. Keep in mind that the foods listed may be changed from year to year, so always be sure to check for the most updated version.

UNCOVERING POSSIBLE FOOD INTOLERANCE

Food intolerance can be an issue for your gut and immune health. Many people get food intolerance and food allergies confused. When you go to the allergist and get a skin prick test or a blood test, they are testing for a true food allergy. Food allergies and food intolerances are common, but a food intolerance test does not show up on an allergy test.

The most common type of food allergy is an IgE-mediated reaction, which can lead to an immediate reaction due to the release of histamine as well as mast cells. Some of the common symptoms of a food allergy include hives, itching, swelling, difficulty breathing, wheezing, and even anaphylaxis in very severe allergic reactions.

Food intolerance, on the other hand, is more common than allergic reactions to foods and does not involve the immune system. With a true food allergy, there is an IgE reaction that is immediate and can cause anaphylactic reactions, throat swelling, and hives. With a food intolerance, there is an IgA and an IgG reaction, which can cause inflammation and produces more diffuse symptoms. The food itself can trigger the intolerance, or your body reacts to the particular food. For example, with lactose intolerance, the body is unable to break down the lactose in dairy products. Another example is a histamine intolerance, where someone may react to histamines in certain foods and respond with a migraine headache. Food intolerance can occur due to a number of factors, including not having the proper enzymes to actually digest the food, having reactions to additives in foods, or being sensitive to certain chemicals or toxins found in certain food products. The symptoms associated with a food intolerance include digestive issues, such as gas, bloating, diarrhea, constipation, and nausea. Food intolerance can occur at any time and to any food. More times than not, it occurs with the foods that we consume most frequently and often the foods that we gravitate toward when we are stressed.

There are a couple of different ways to test for food intolerance. There are blood tests generally offered through functional medicine practitioners, and these test for specific food intolerance. This is the definitive way of knowing what you are truly sensitive to. If you suspect you may be intolerant to a specific food, you can also try an elimination diet by completely removing it from your diet for at least two weeks and then reintroducing it and seeing how you feel. Keep in mind that if you have a true food allergy, these foods should never be reintroduced into the diet.

HEALING WITH THE PALEO-STYLE DIETARY APPROACH

Once we determine which foods you are intolerant to, we can determine which dietary approach will work best. I recommend a paleo-style approach when healing from Hashimoto's; however, if there are foods that are paleo–approved that you are sensitive to, they would not be included in your particular dietary protocol. There are also some paleo-approved foods that I still don't recommend someone add into their diet. Each person is going to be different, and everyone has a different level of sensitivity to certain foods. Some may have none, while others may have a handful. Working around these in a way to make it work for you is the best approach to heal your gut and your thyroid.

The paleo-style diet approach is what I recommend long–term after the initial 30-Day Thyroid Reset. The paleo diet eliminates the most commonly reactive foods as a way to reduce the inflammatory response in the body and thus help promote healing. Reducing the inflammatory response is an essential part in getting into remission, because inflammation is at the root of autoimmune diseases like Hashimoto's.

THE 30-DAY THYROID RESET

What follows are more specific dietary protocols that I often suggest for my patients to help them get on the right track and feel better. Let's take a look at what the first initial 30-Day Thyroid Reset looks like.

It's important to remember that this thyroid reset isn't about fasting or losing weight, so don't get hung up on tracking ratios or how many calories you are taking in versus how many you are burning. The point of this diet is literally just as it sounds. It's a reset to help reduce the inflammatory response in your body and help get you on a healthier track for healthier thyroid function.

Clean 15

1. Sweet corn
2. Avocados
3. Pineapple
4. Cabbage
5. Onions
6. Sweet peas, frozen
7. Papayas
8. Asparagus
9. Mangos
10. Eggplant
11. Honeydew melon
12. Kiwi
13. Cantaloupe
14. Cauliflower
15. Grapefruit

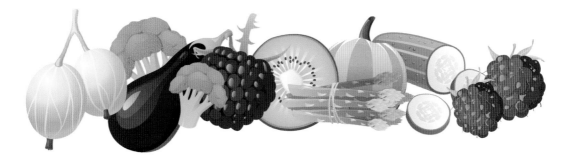

Dirty Dozen

1. Strawberries
2. Spinach
3. Nectarines
4. Apples
5. Peaches
6. Pears
7. Cherries
8. Grapes
9. Celery
10. Tomatoes
11. Sweet bell and hot peppers
12. Potatoes

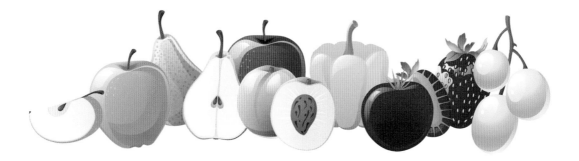

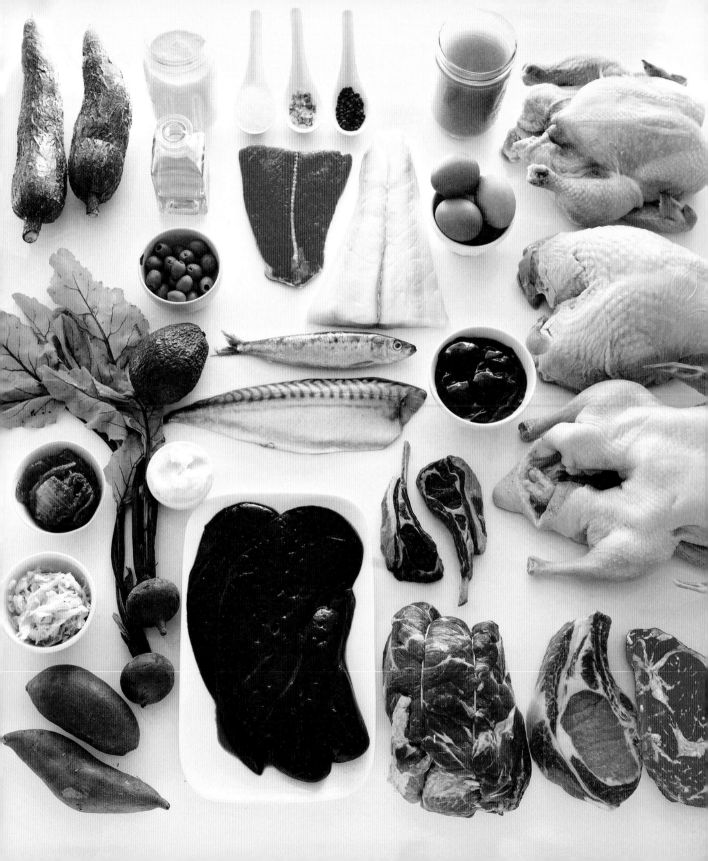

WHAT WILL YOU BE EATING?

The foods are split up into different categories: foods that you can enjoy without restrictions, foods you should limit, and foods that you should completely keep out of your diet.

EAT WITHOUT RESTRICTIONS: Enjoy these foods as you see fit!

LIMIT THESE FOODS: Watch how much you consume. If a food is on this list, it doesn't mean you have to completely eliminate it from your diet, but do limit your intake.

KEEP OUT OF YOUR DIET: Completely eliminate these foods from your diet. These foods will get in the way of your body's healing ability on the thyroid reset, and they should be avoided after the reset portion of the diet is complete as well.

EAT WITHOUT RESTRICTIONS

ORGANIC AND FREE-RANGE ANIMAL PRODUCTS: I emphasize organic and free-range here because it's especially important during this critical 30-day reset period. You do not want to be exposing your body to harmful hormones, antibiotics, or steroids found in conventional animal products. Focus on beef and lamb. Pork, turkey, chicken, duck, and venison are also good options.

ORGAN MEATS: Liver is especially great during the 30-day reset.

FREE-RANGE AND ORGANIC EGGS

WILD-CAUGHT FISH: Fish high in healthy omega-3 fatty acids such as salmon, herring, and mackerel are excellent choices. Get three servings of fatty fish in your diet per week at 6 ounces (180 g) each.

BONE BROTH: Bone broth is packed full of nutrition, is rich in amino acids and glycine and is excellent for gut health. You can add liver and other organ meats to bone broth to make a delicious soup.

STARCHY VEGETABLES: You will want to focus on tubers here, such as sweet potatoes, yams, yuca, and taro. *Note:* Refer to the section on goitrogens to learn about adding things like yuca and sweet potatoes into your diet.

NON-STARCHY VEGETABLES: You can enjoy these both cooked and raw and focus on fermented options that will help promote gut health. Sauerkraut, kimchi, beets, and coconut kefir are good choices.

HEALTHY FATS: Coconut oil, olive oil, palm oil, lard, duck fat, beef tallow, olives, avocados, and coconut milk are all good options.

SPICES: Instead of seasoning with sugar and refined salt, opt for sea salt and organic spices.

LIMIT THESE FOODS

PROCESSED MEAT: Significantly reduce or even keep processed meats out of your diet, especially the ones that contain gluten, sugar, and soy. If you do consume some processed meat options such as sausage and bacon, purchase organic, free-range, and nitrate-free options and enjoy in moderation during the 30-Day Thyroid Reset. You will find some recipes that contain sausage and bacon in the recipe section of this book, so be sure to get a paleo-friendly, organic, and nitrate-free option.

CERTAIN FRUITS: Keep fruit intake low to no more than three servings per day. If you have difficulty balancing your blood sugar levels, limit your intake even further to either one serving per day or eliminate it altogether. Choose lower sugar fruits such as berries over higher sugar options like apples. See the fructose chart on page 73.

NUTS AND SEEDS: During the 30-Day Thyroid Reset, soak nuts for at least 12 hours and then dehydrate before eating. This will help you better absorb the nuts and seeds, but keep your intake to a handful or less per day. You will find a homemade almond milk recipe in the recipe section that uses soaked almonds.

CAFFEINE: Caffeinated beverages such as coffee and black tea should be enjoyed in moderation during the 30-day reset period. If you do have a cup of tea or coffee in the morning, enjoy it with a splash of full-fat coconut milk instead of heavy cream. Caffeine should only be consumed early on in the day before lunchtime and should be kept to one cup or less. If you suffer from low blood sugar, difficulty sleeping, or even chronic fatigue, caffeine should be completely eliminated.

MISCELLANEOUS FOOD ITEMS: If you do want chocolate, you can have very small amounts of 70 percent or darker dark chocolate as long as it's unsweetened. Apple cider vinegar can be had in moderation if you enjoy adding vinegar to your cooking.

DINING OUT: There are too many unhealthy food options available in restaurants, so keep dining out limited during the 30-day reset period and make most of your food at home. When you cook at home, you are in charge of the foods that go into your dish, so you can be sure you are following the reset diet as closely as possible. This is extremely important during the first 30 days!

Fructose Chart

Fruit	Serving Size	Grams of Fructose
Lime	1 medium	0
Lemon	1 medium	0.6
Cranberry	1 cup (100 g)	0.7
Passion Fruit	1 medium	0.9
Prune	1 medium	1.2
Apricot	1 medium	1.3
Guava	2 medium	2.2
Date (Deglet Noor)	1 medium	2.6
Cantaloupe	⅛ medium melon	2.8
Raspberry	1 cup (123 g)	3.0
Clemetine	1 medium	3.4
Kiwifruit	1 medium	3.4
Blackberry	1 cup (144 g)	3.5
Star Fruit	1 medium	3.6
Cherry, Sweet	10	3.8
Strawberry	1 cup (151 g)	3.8
Cherry, Sour	1 cup (138 g)	4.0
Pineapple	3.5" x 7.5" slice (9 × 20 cm)	4.0
Grapefruit	½ medium	4.3
Boysenberry	1 cup (132 g)	4.6
Tangerine/Mandarin	1 medium	4.8
Nectarine	1 medium	5.4
Peach	1 medium	5.9
Navel Orange	1 medium	6.1
Papaya	½ medium	6.3
Honeydew	⅛ medium	6.7
Banana	1 medium	7.1
Blueberry	1 cup (148 g)	7.4
Apple	1 medium	7.6
Date (Medjool)	1 medium	7.7
Persimmon	1 medium	10.6
Watermelon	1/16 medium	11.3
Pear	1 medium	11.8
Raisin	¼ cup (40 g)	12.3
Grape, Seedless	1 cup (151 g)	12.4
Mango	½ medium	16.2
Aprictot, Dried	1 cup (190 g)	16.4
Fig, Dried	1 cup (149 g)	23.0

Have only 10 g or less of fructose a day. The fruits in red should be avoided.
Source: www.mercola.com.

KEEP OUT OF YOUR DIET

DAIRY PRODUCTS: All dairy, including goat and sheep products, should be kept out of your diet during the 30-day reset.

AVOID

- Yogurt
- Butter
- Cheese
- Milk
- Ghee
- Heavy cream
- Sour cream
- Whey

SUGAR: Avoid all natural and artificial sugars. Even natural sugar such as pure maple syrup, honey, brown rice syrup, and agave should be kept out of your diet during the 30-day reset. Avoid any high fructose corn syrup (HFCS) during and after the reset, as HFCS is extremely damaging to your health. Artificial sweeteners should also be completely eliminated and kept out of the diet long–term.

WATCH OUT FOR TERMS LIKE

- Erythritol
- Mannitol
- Sorbitol
- Xylitol
- Aspartame
- Equal
- Splenda
- Sucralose
- NutraSweet
- Sweet'n Low
- Sugar
- Brown sugar
- Honey
- Agave
- Molasses
- Barley
- Malt
- Cane sugar
- Coconut sugar
- Malt syrup
- Sucrose
- Rice syrup
- Brown rice syrup
- Refined sugar
- Raw sugar
- Evaporated cane juice
- Corn sweetener
- Corn syrup
- Date sugar
- Dehydrated cane juice
- Dextrose
- Glucose
- Galactose
- High fructose corn syrup
- Monk fruit
- Palm sugar

SUGARY BEVERAGES: Avoid any beverage that is not water! Soda and fruit juices, both diet and regular, should be avoided. Alcohol should also be avoided during the 30-day reset.

PROCESSED FOODS: These are foods that are best to keep out of your diet even after the first 30-day reset. After 30 days without them, you will wonder why you ever ate them to begin with because you will feel so good without them in your diet! Stick to whole foods versus foods that are packaged or frozen. Even some of the common foods that get marked as "healthy" like certain protein powders and energy bars are still processed and contain unneeded chemicals. Be sure to steer clear of processed foods and go for foods in their whole and natural state, such as meats, fish, fruits, and vegetables. Keep in mind that in the thyroid reset I recommend an unsweetened collagen protein powder, which is different than other protein powders that may come with lots of unnecessary ingredients.

Here are some of the added ingredients to watch out for when looking at food labels, to make sure what you buy is as unprocessed as possible:

- Brominated vegetable oil
- Lecithin
- Hydrolyzed vegetable protein
- Monosodium glutamate
- Nitrates
- Nitrites
- Textured vegetable protein
- Hydrogenated or partially hydrogenated vegetable oils
- Yeast extract
- Artificial flavors
- Natural flavors
- Artificial food dyes

DAMAGED OILS: Not all oils are created equal, and there are many damaged oils that should be kept out of your diet long after the first 30 days. Stay away from soybean, corn, canola, cottonseed, sunflower, and safflower oils. These are processed vegetable oils that are very high in omega-6 fatty acids and should be eliminated from the diet. Coconut oil is a great option, especially for cooking, due to its high smoke point, and extra virgin olive oil makes a great salad dressing or marinade.

GLUTEN: Gluten is particularly bad for anyone who suffers from a thyroid condition. The body can mistake a protein in gluten as part of the thyroid and thus initiate an attack on the thyroid itself. When your body is already attacking your own thyroid tissue, this is obviously not something you want to happen. Gluten is also very hard to digest and causes inflammation in the body. It's important to go entirely gluten-free and avoid anything containing barley, rye, and wheat.

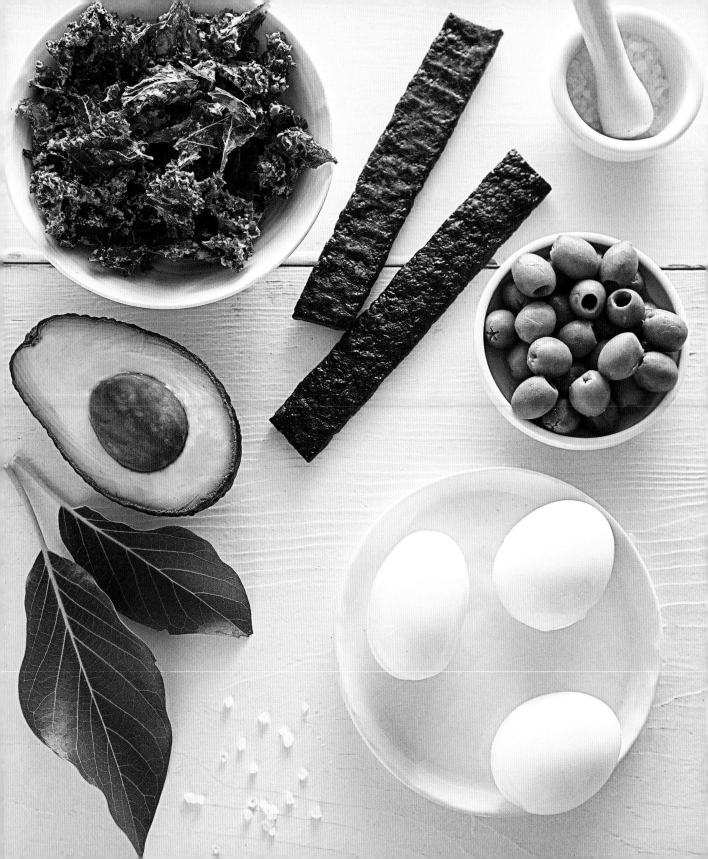

GRAINS: All grains should be removed from the diet. This goes for pseudo-grains and gluten-free grains such as quinoa.

AVOID ALL GRAINS, INCLUDING

- Barley
- Corn
- Durum
- Millet
- Kamut
- Rice

- Rye
- Spelt
- Teff
- Wheat
- Oats

LEGUMES: Avoid all legumes and beans.

CERTAIN SAUCES AND SPICES: Anything that is packaged is suspect. Avoid any packaged seasonings because they often contain sugar, corn, and gluten. Also avoid soy sauce and any other bottled sauces. You will find that there are plenty of healthy ways to season your food that don't involve any processed products and that taste better and are so much better for you!

ALCOHOL: While the occasional glass of wine may be OK after a healing diet has been incorporated for a period of time, keep alcohol out of your diet most of the time and completely out of your diet during the first 30 days.

A NOTE ABOUT SNACKS

If you find that you are hungry between meals, here are some easy grab-and-go options:

- Grass-fed beef sticks
- Kale chips
- Olives

- Hard-boiled eggs (not for Option 2; see page 89)
- Avocados with sea salt

To make things easier for you, a sample 30-day meal plan and accompanying shopping lists are on pages 178 and 179.

DR. CAMPBELL'S FAVORITE SUPERFOODS

A handful of superfoods are some of my favorite options to include in a healing protocol. Keep in mind that not all of them will be appropriate for the 30-Day Thyroid Reset, but many of my patients have been able to enjoy most if not all of these superfoods after the thyroid reset. These are good nutrient-dense foods to keep in mind. Most can be included in the diet after the reset, if not during the reset itself. The full-fat raw dairy in particular is something that should be avoided until you are advised to add it back into your diet.

SEAWEED: Seaweed is one of my favorite paleo superfoods because it is packed full of minerals and provides your body with unique nutrients that many other foods do not offer.

DARK LEAFY GREEN VEGETABLES: Vegetables are an essential part of a healthy diet, and dark leafy greens pack in a healthy dose of vitamins and minerals. Some of my favorite options include kale, collard greens, and spinach.

ORGAN MEATS: Organ meats are certainly not as commonly enjoyed as other parts of the animal, but they make their way onto my list of favorite superfoods because they are packed with essential vitamins. Organ meat does take some getting used to; when cooked in soups and stews, it's not only nourishing but delicious as well. I also want to mention that if you absolutely cannot tolerate the taste of liver, you don't have to eat it. I often get asked this by many of my patients, and while I stress how great it is for overall health, it is not required that you eat it. You will, however, find chicken liver in the thyroid reset recipes. I encourage you to give it a try, and if you cannot tolerate it, then I recommend you simply swap it with an organic chicken breast.

WILD-CAUGHT FISH: Wild-caught, fatty fish provides the body with the omega-3 fatty acids EPA and DHA, which are powerful anti-inflammatory fatty acids, and they are essential for heart health. Some good, low-mercury choices include wild-caught salmon, sardines, mackerel, and herring. Aim to consume some fatty fish about three times per week or a total of 1 pound (455 g) per week.

ORGANIC PASTURE-RAISED EGGS: Eggs are one of nature's most nutrient-dense foods. One single egg holds 13 essential nutrients. Many people believe that eggs are only healthy if you consume the egg white, but all the nutrition is in the yolk, so be sure to eat the entire egg as part of your diet. If eggs are well-tolerated, you can consume them daily.

FERMENTED FOODS: Fermented foods are excellent for gut health, and as you now know, a large part of healing from Hashimoto's involves taking care of your digestive system and boosting healthy gut flora. Fermented foods are rich in probiotics, so be sure to include them in your diet. Sauerkraut, kimchi, and unsweetened coconut yogurt are all great options.

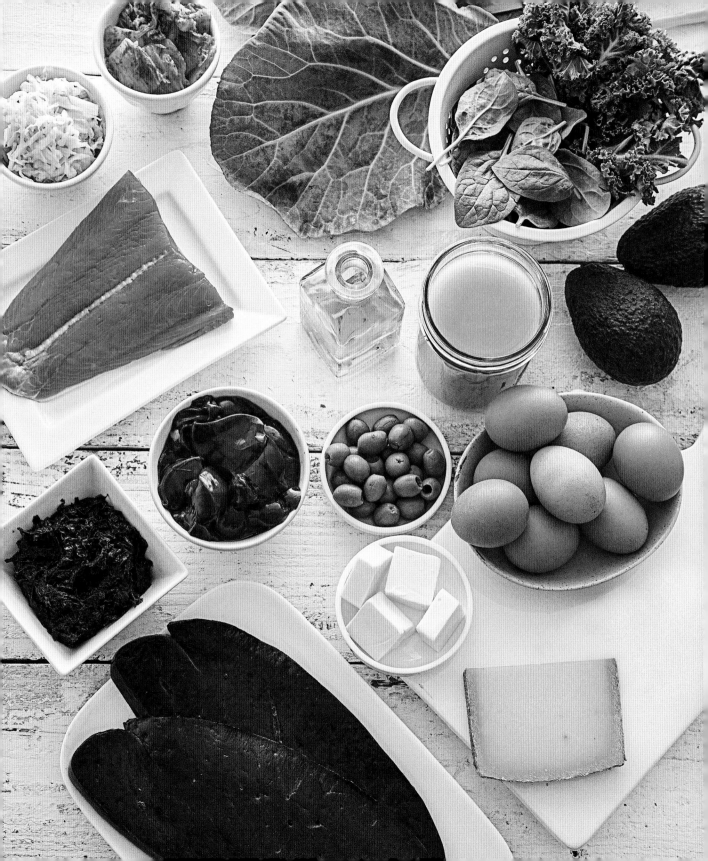

GRASS-FED, RAW, FULL-FAT DAIRY: This is the one superfood on the list that should be included after the initial reset and should only be included if symptoms have significantly improved. With that being said, if tolerated, full-fat raw, grass-fed dairy can provide the body with some significant health benefits. It is a rich source of fat-soluble vitamins such as A, D, and K2 and is, of course, rich in calcium. It's also a great source of healthy bacteria and conjugated linoleic acid (CLA). Cheeses made from raw milk can be found in many natural foods stores and online. Raw milk is available in some states, so this may be more accessible to some than others, depending on where you live. Refer to the reintroduction section for more on casein and auto-immune disease.

HEALTHY FATS: Fats are essential for overall health, but unfortunately in today's society so many people have been told to avoid fat in order to protect heart health. The truth is that the body needs a certain amount of fat to function, and as long as it's in the form of healthy options it can actually be very beneficial for your overall health. Focus on ghee and grass-fed butter if dairy is tolerated, coconut oil, olives and olive oil, avocados, palm oil, lard, and even duck fat. The great thing about these healthy fats is that they may actually help lower your triglyceride levels while raising your HDL cholesterol levels (the good kind of cholesterol) and can also help with your energy levels as well. Try to get 2 to 4 tablespoons (30 to 60 ml) of these healthy fats into your diet each day.

BONE BROTH: One of the most popular paleo superfoods at the moment is bone broth. While bone broth has just recently stepped into the spotlight for its superfood qualities, it has been around for many years. Think about it, when you were growing up and came down with a cold, did your grandmother ever make you homemade chicken noodle soup? Chances are it was using a homemade stock. These homemade stocks and broths can actually help boost the immune system and protect the body. Bone broth is rich in amino acids and minerals and is highly absorbable in the body. It's also excellent for gut health and for those who suffer from leaky gut, which most people with autoimmune disease do. I recommend that my patients consume bone broth daily.

THE RAW MILK DIFFERENCE

I want to touch upon something important when it comes to dairy. When I talk about being able to potentially reintroduce dairy (only if tolerated), I am specifically talking about raw milk, ghee, and grass-fed butter. I thought it was important to share exactly why raw dairy is different from conventional products, so let's dive deeper into that.

There are different proteins present in cow's milk, with casein being the one I am going to talk about here. In older breeds of cows referred to as A2 cows, the beta-casein present contains proline, which is an amino acid. However, in A1 cows, the proline turns into histidine through mutation. This will become important, so keep reading! Another important fact is that beta-casein contains B-casomorphin-7, also known as BCM-7, which has been linked to gastrointestinal effects similar to what occurs in those with lactose intolerance. BCM-7 also acts as a naturally occurring opiate. Yes, you heard that right. What is found in conventional milk has opiate-like properties.

Now, remember those older cows known as A2 cows? As it turns out, the proline present in these cows is able to keep the BCM-7 out of the milk because of a bond it has with this particular protein. This bond helps keep the BCM-7 out of the cow's system. However, the A1 cows are not able to keep the BCM-7 out because it contains histidine, which has a very weak hold on BCM-7, allowing it to get into the milk and then into anyone who ingests it.

The thing about dairy production in the United States is that A1 cows are used for most of the dairy products you find in stores. The scary part is that milk from A1 cows that contains large amounts of BCM-7 has been linked to autoimmune disease, which is the last thing we want when trying to repair and support thyroid health.

This information is crucial to keep in mind when I talk about reintroducing certain dairy products (see page 87). If, and only if, your body tolerates dairy, it must be raw and specifically labeled as A2 milk. Depending on the state that you live in, certain health and wellness stores sell raw A2 milk that is clearly labeled. Remember that A2 raw milk does not come with the same side effects as A1 milk for a lot of people. In fact, one study shows that the consumption of milk that contained A1 B-casein was linked to gastrointestinal inflammation as well as a decrease in cognitive processing speed. However, drinking A2 B-casein milk did not cause any type of issues in people with post-dairy digestive discomfort, both those who had a lactose intolerance and those who did not.

The bottom line is that if your body does tolerate dairy, be sure to stick to raw A2 milk and grass-fed butter or ghee. However, keep in mind that those with Hashimoto's may not be able to tolerate any dairy, including raw dairy, so don't be discouraged if this is not something that you are able to tolerate. Everyone is different, and it will all depend on your tolerance after you go through the 30-Day Thyroid Reset Plan.

SMOOTHIES

During the thyroid reset, you will find a handful of smoothie recipes to incorporate into your diet. I absolutely love smoothies for a number of reasons. For one, they are quick and simple to make and two, it is very easy to pack in a powerful dose of nutritional value in a single meal when you add superfoods to your smoothies.

I want to talk about some of the superfoods you will find in the smoothies during the reset and why they are going to be so beneficial for your health.

AVOCADOS: Adding avocados to smoothies is an excellent way to bulk it up and give it a little more substance to keep you feeling full for longer periods of time. Avocados add a creamy consistency, and they are also a great source of healthy fat, fiber, and magnesium.

PLANTAINS: I love adding plantains to recipes whenever possible because they are an excellent source of resistant starch. Why is this important? Patients with thyroid conditions require carbohydrates in order to convert T4 into T3, and the resistant starch present in the plantains helps feed the good bacteria in the gut. Remember that the majority of our immune system lives in our gut, so it's essential that we feed our gut with foods to support overall health.

COCONUT BUTTER: You will find this superfood in many of the smoothie recipes because it's an excellent way to add some healthy fat into each smoothie while also adding a delicious tropical flavor. Healthy fats are important for overall health, and they are rich in lauric acid, which helps support the immune system. This is critical when trying to address an autoimmune condition.

YOUNG COCONUT MEAT: Young coconut meat is the flesh of green coconuts, and it's rich in dietary fiber, healthy fats, and B vitamins and helps keep your body hydrated.

HOMEMADE ALMOND MILK: I love almond milk, but unfortunately the almond milk you would buy from the store is often filled with unnecessary ingredients. During the thyroid reset, you will find a very simple homemade vanilla almond milk recipe that you can easily include in your smoothie recipes. The recipe is made with everything your body needs and nothing it doesn't!

COCONUT MILK: You will also find coconut milk as the base liquid for many of these smoothie recipes. Just like the other coconut products listed here, coconut milk is packed full of healthy fats and also makes for an incredibly creamy and filling smoothie. It's also used when almond milk is not well-tolerated or if you choose to follow the additional 30-day diet after the initial reset. Coconut milk is also a great milk to start with if you are just beginning to eliminate dairy from your diet because it's one of the creamiest nondairy milk options.

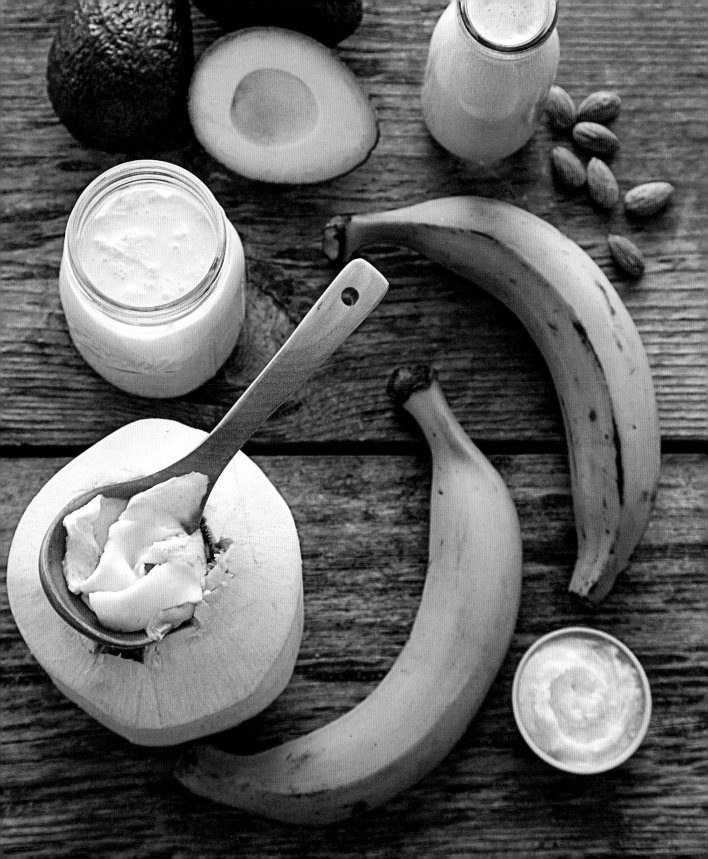

So, after all that smoothie talk, I bet you are ready to get started. But how do you make the perfect smoothie?

Many people think it's just about tossing all the ingredients into the blender and blending it up 1-2-3, and that's not entirely wrong. You can blend everything up without adding the ingredients in any particular order; however, there is a science behind making the perfect smoothie. This is the easiest and best way I have found to make the creamiest and smoothest smoothie yet.

How to Make the
Perfect Smoothie

Step 1 **Add the liquid:**

This is almond milk or coconut milk.

Step 3 **Add the fruits and veggies:**

Next, add your fruits and vegetables other than the ones used as your base. Berries and spinach should now be added.

Step 2 **Add the base:**

This makes your smoothie creamy. Avocados, plantains, and bananas should be added here.

Step 4 **Add in superfoods:**

This includes flax seeds, chia seeds, coconut butter, and protein powders.

Step 5 **Blend:**

The last step is to just blend it up! Each smoothie will require different blending times depending on how thick the smoothie is. You will likely need to blend for 30 to 60 seconds, and if your blender comes with a tamper, you may need to use that to push all the ingredients down.

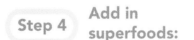

WHAT YOU NEED TO KNOW ABOUT GOITROGENS DURING THE RESET

This list is specifically for those who have actually been diagnosed with a thyroid condition, so if you have not been diagnosed this list may not pertain to you but may be useful if you want to learn more about goitrogenic foods.

Goitrogenic foods have received a bad reputation among those who suffer from thyroid conditions, but the truth is that completely avoiding these foods may not be entirely necessary. Cooking these foods significantly helps reduce their goitrogenic effect. The foods on this list are things you may not wish to consume daily, but in moderation they are nutritious.

The problem thyroid patients may have with goitrogenic foods is that goitrogens can actually reduce the uptake of iodine by the thyroid gland, but this can be fixed with proper iodine intake. As I have previously mentioned, I much prefer to recommend that my patients get their iodine from food sources such as seaweed or kelp flakes than in supplemental form. Thyroid patients will want to continue to keep some goitrogenic foods in their diet because they do offer some health benefits, but you will want to avoid large intakes.

As far as consuming these raw, you should be able to do so in moderation as long as your iodine intake is up to par, but this rule does not apply to mothers who are breastfeeding. Breastfeeding moms should reduce their consumption of raw cruciferous veggies to make sure that there is enough iodine in their milk. They can also increase iodine-rich foods in their diet with things like seaweed.

A NOTE ABOUT SWEET POTATOES AND YUCA

In the 30-Day Thyroid Reset, you will find sweet potatoes and yuca as part of the dietary plan, and I know that many people with thyroid diseases may question why there are goitrogenic foods in the thyroid reset. To better help explain the goitrogen and thyroid connection I want to share the importance of consuming starchy carbohydrates.

Sweet potatoes and yuca are lightly goitrogenic, but thyroid patients need starchy carbohydrates in their diet for the conversion of T4 into T3, so I do encourage patients to consume these. Cooking these starchy vegetables helps them lose their goitrogenic effect. It's important to have these two as staples in your diet and to not avoid them solely for the fact that they have goitrogenic properties. With proper cooking, they are normally very well-tolerated and beneficial for thyroid patients, especially when you don't overdo it.

Goitrogens

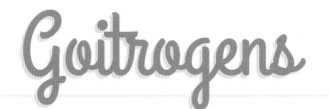

CRUCIFEROUS VEGETABLES	OTHER FOODS
Bok choy	Bamboo shoots
Broccoli	Cassava (yuca)
Broccolini	Millet
Brussels sprouts	Peaches
Cabbage	Peanuts
Canola/Rapeseed	Pears
Cauliflower	Pine nuts
Chinese cabbage	Soybeans (tofu, soybean oil, soy protein isolate, soy lecithin)
Choy sum	Spinach
Collard greens	Strawberries
Horseradish	Sweet potatoes
Kai-lan	
Kale	
Mizuna	
Mustard greens and seeds	
Radish	
Rapini	
Rutabaga	
Tatsoi	
Turnip	

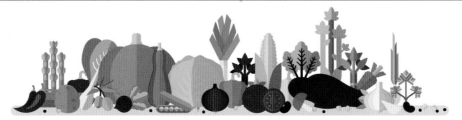

AFTER THE FIRST 30 DAYS

After you make it through the first 30 days, then what? For most patients, the 30-day reset is followed by a two-week reintroduction plan, but for some patients with autoimmune conditions, a 30-day reset may not be enough. In this case, I like to do another 30 days where nightshades, eggs, and nuts are also eliminated. Once symptoms start to get better, some patients can begin adding dairy back into their diet as well as eggs, nuts, and nightshades, but gluten is never added back in.

Here are the steps to take after the initial 30–day reset. Keep in mind that each patient will be different:

OPTION 1: If you did well with the first 30 days, you can jump right into the two-week reintroduction diet.

OPTION 2: If you are still having symptoms, continue with another 30 days on the reset plan, but also eliminate eggs, peppers, tomatoes, potatoes, eggplant, and nuts.

OPTION 1: TWO-WEEK REINTRODUCTION DIET

If you are following Option 1 after the initial 30-Day Thyroid Reset, that means that you are feeling better! That's an amazing thing and something to be proud of. Thus far, you have been keeping certain foods such as dairy out of your diet, but during the two-week reintroduction, we start to reintroduce things like raw dairy and raw honey. This two-week reintroduction diet should be taken slowly.

When you slowly reintroduce foods, it's easier for you to determine which foods are going to agree with your body and which are not. Another reason for adding foods back into your diet is that many of the foods not allowed on the 30-day reset are nutrient-dense and can help your body heal once you reset. You want to nourish your body with the highest quality foods possible, so adding some of the foods back in if well–tolerated is usually beneficial. One of the foods I like to reintroduce into a patient's diet is dairy in the form of raw and grass-fed dairy products. Conventional dairy should continue to stay out of the diet because it is packed with hormones, antibiotics, and steroids. However, raw dairy may hold some important health benefits for those with autoimmune diseases. Raw milk has been shown to help boost glutathione levels, which is helpful for the immune system.

This stage of the diet is the most challenging because symptoms may not return for hours, days, or even weeks after consuming a particular food, which can make pinpointing reactive foods tricky. Some patients may have very strong and immediate reactions, while others may have delayed reactions or symptoms that aren't noticeable enough to pinpoint origins. Keep in mind that if a true food allergy is present, that food should never be reintroduced.

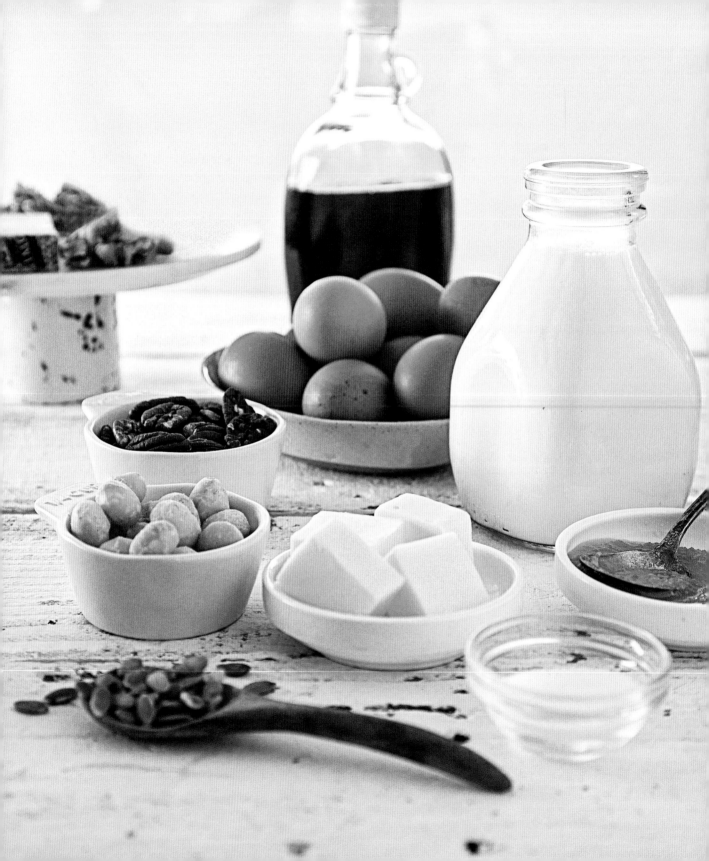

Reintroduce one food at a time for three days straight before moving on to the next food item. The immune system can take some time to react and cause any noticeable symptoms when dealing with a food sensitivity. Keep an eye out for any symptoms you would commonly associate with your autoimmune condition or things like fatigue and digestive upset. If symptoms do occur, keep that food out of your diet.

It's also a little more complicated than just reintroducing foods in whatever order you choose. For example, when reintroducing dairy, do so in a specific order. Start with ghee, which contains a small amount of milk protein, followed by things like butter, yogurt, kefir, cheese, and then raw milk. Starting with the dairy product that has the lowest amount of milk protein can help uncover a potential reaction before you overdo it.

Here is a list of foods that can be reintroduced during this two-week period. The ultimate goal is to eventually consume a paleo-style diet with a small amount of raw dairy if tolerated.

- Raw dairy
- Grass-fed butter
- Grade B pure maple syrup
- Raw honey
- Stevia
- Soaked nuts

OPTION 2: ADDITIONAL 30-DAY DIET

If you have chosen Option 2 that means you are still experiencing some symptoms. I cannot stress how important it is for you not to get discouraged! Keep in mind that your body has likely been in an inflammatory state for a long period of time—perhaps years. It can take time for you to feel completely better, and for some people it will be necessary to do an additional 30-day diet. This time eliminate eggs, nightshade vegetables (peppers, tomatoes, potatoes, eggplant), and nuts, and continue to keep out dairy. This is very similar to the first 30 days, but this time around you are following some stricter guidelines.

After another 30 days of following the thyroid reset minus the eggs, dairy, nightshade vegetables, and nuts you can then try the two-week reintroduction diet. To help get you started, I have adjusted the 30-Day Thyroid Reset for you to use during an additional 30 days for those of you who need to continue with this protocol and watch the diet even more closely for potentially reactive foods. Follow the same thyroid reset but pay attention to the * on the Meal Plan on page 178 because it will serve as your guide for this additional 30-day diet.

GOING PALEO

Now that you have completed the 30-Day Thyroid Reset and possibly an additional 30 days after that, it's time to talk about the long-term approach to combatting Hashimoto's.

As I have talked about throughout this book, I recommend a paleo-style approach as the long-term dietary goal with some thyroid-specific variations. In this chapter, we are going to explore how you can uncover possible food sensitivities and work around them when following a paleo diet. A "going paleo cheat sheet" will help you jump into a paleo-style diet without stress.

Paleo Cheat Sheet

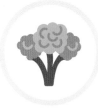

Vegetables

All organic vegetables except corn, peas, white potatoes

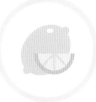

Fruits

All organic low-sugar fruits, no-sugar added dried fruits

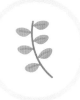

Fresh Herbs

All organic fresh herbs

Dried Herbs and Spices

All spices and dried herbs without any added ingredients, sea salt and Himalayan pink sea salt

Healthy Fats and Oils

Extra virgin or extra light tasting olive oil, coconut oil, avocado oil

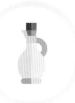

Condiments

Sugar-free Dijon mustard, paleo-style mayonnaise, although this is best if made homemade, vinegar except for rice vinegar

Seafood

All fish except tilapia and best if wild-caught

Baking Items

Almond and coconut flour, unsweetened shredded coconut, pure vanilla beans, raw unsweetened cocoa powder

Sweeteners

Pure grade B maple syrup, raw honey

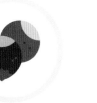

Nuts and Seeds

All raw or sprouted nuts and seeds, no-sugar-added nut butters with no other added ingredients, tahini, nut milks are best homemade but you can have store-bought, sugar-free nut milks that are also free from carrageenan

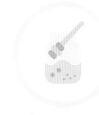

Meat, Poultry, Eggs

Beef, best if grass-fed; bison, best if grass-fed; pork, chicken, turkey; eggs, best if pasture-raised and organic

DR. CAMPBELL'S FAVORITE STORE-BOUGHT PALEO PRODUCTS

Let's face it: life's busy, and there may be a time where you need to grab a snack on the go or just don't have time to make everything from scratch. While I recommend making as much as you can, especially during the initial 30-day reset period, it's also OK to pick up some paleo-friendly things at the store after the reset and once you have your symptoms really under control.

I have listed some of my favorite places to purchase these paleo-friendly foods and then some of my favorite options as well.

ONLINE WHOLESALE STORE: Thrive Market

Thrive Market offers abundant, affordable paleo-friendly foods that you can order and have delivered straight to your door! I highly recommend this site to anyone who is looking to save some money or doesn't have a health food store local to them, as Thrive offers just about any paleo grab-and-go option.

FAVORITE PALEO PACKAGED AND PREPARED FOODS

GRASS-FED JERKY: EPIC bars, Tanka Bars, Primal Pacs

BARS: Go Raw, YAWP

NUT BUTTERS: Artisana, Once Again

OTHER SNACKS: Lydia's organic kale chips, Honest sweet potato chips, Tropical Traditional olives, GimMe seaweed snacks, Tropical Traditional coconut products

PREPARED MEATS: US Wellness, Butcher Box

CANNED FISH: Vital Choice, Wild Planet

YOGURT AND KEFIR: Maple Hill Creamery, Blue Hill

CONDIMENTS: Primal Kitchen

BREAD, BAGEL, AND PANCAKE MIXES: Legit Bread Company

CRACKERS, COOKIES, MUFFINS, AND CAKE MIXES: Simple Mills

GOING PALEO ON A BUDGET

Starting any new diet can be pricey, and going paleo can certainly increase your grocery bill if you are not careful. This doesn't mean that you can't eat a paleo-style diet when on a budget; in fact, it's easy to do so. With some modifications to shopping lists and a little meal prep, you can very realistically keep your grocery bill reasonable when switching over to a paleo way of eating. Here are some tips to help you go paleo on a budget.

BUY CONVENTIONAL SOMETIMES: Eating organic whenever you possibly can is best, but it can be expensive. It's OK to cut corners when needed. If it's just not in your budget to buy everything organic, try to stick to organic when purchasing foods that have the most contamination, and then go conventional if you need to for the foods that are least contaminated. This will save you quite a bit of money each time you go shopping.

BUY IN BULK: If you don't have a membership to a warehouse store, it may be worth investing in one because it can save you a large chunk of money when it comes to your grocery bill. Organic coconut oil, nuts, and seeds are much cheaper when purchased in bulk. Think about investing in a membership to one of these stores to save you money in the long run.

BUY ONLINE: Believe it or not, there are stores online now that offer lower prices than your grocery store may offer. Amazon even offers something called Amazon Pantry where you can buy dry goods for a fraction of the cost of some grocery store items. Thrive Market is another excellent option. For a membership fee, you can find all sorts of paleo-friendly foods at a very reasonable price online. If you buy your dry goods online and your produce and meat at a grocery store you may be surprised at how much money you can save.

MENU PLANNING: Although menu planning may seem like a pain, it can be very beneficial for your health as well as your wallet! If you plan meals for an entire month, you can make multiple meals using the same ingredients to keep costs down.

BATCH COOK: When you batch cook, you save yourself time during the week, and you can also save yourself some money. Think about slow cooker recipes you want to make for the week and prep them all ahead of time and then freeze them. Batch cooking also allows you to use some of the same ingredients for each recipe to help keep costs down.

KEEP IT SIMPLE: It's easy to get carried away and go for the most extravagant items available, but that's not necessary. Stick to the basics of meats, fruits, veggies, nuts, and seeds to keep your costs down and to also fuel your body right.

SKIP BOXED ITEMS: Many companies are now marketing their products as paleo–friendly, but that's not necessarily always the case, and they aren't always healthy, either. These products also tend to be very pricey, so staying away from packaged items will save you money.

STOCK UP ON SALES: If organic chicken or grass-fed beef is on sale one week, stock up! You can always freeze what you don't plan to use right away, and it's a great way to save yourself some money.

USE COUPONS: You would be surprised at how many stores offer coupons, and they are basically free money! Take advantage of weekly deals. Many stores also have reward systems where when you rack up a certain amount of points you get money off of your order.

BUY IN SEASON: Purchasing produce in season is a great way to save some money and consume the freshest options available. Going to your local farmers' market is also an excellent way to save some money. Buy lots of fruits and veggies while they are in season and find creative ways to integrate them into your diet.

GROW YOUR OWN: If you have the garden space to grow your own fruits, vegetables, and herbs, go for it! You can save yourself lots of money plus you can ensure that you are consuming the freshest produce available.

BUY FROZEN WHEN NEEDED: In the dead of winter when certain fruits or vegetables just aren't in season, it's OK to buy frozen. I recommend organic frozen fruits and vegetables.

MAKE YOUR OWN CONDIMENTS: Condiments can be expensive, especially the ones specifically marketed as paleo-friendly. Instead of purchasing them at the store, try making your own. You can make your own homemade mayo with just a handful of ingredients using eggs, lemon juice, olive oil, and Dijon mustard. You can also make your own homemade salad dressings to save yourself money. Making your own condiments is also a much healthier option than buying them from the store as you get to decide what you put into each recipe.

PARTICIPATE IN CSA PROGRAMS: Community supported agriculture (CSA) is a great way to get local produce and also save some money on your grocery bill. To get started you must buy a share of a local farm production before the season begins. You can decide how to get local produce delivered to you, how often, and how much you want. This is also a great way to try new and exciting fruits and vegetables.

While starting any new diet can come with some added expenses, with a few adjustments to how you currently grocery shop you will be surprised at how much money you save.

Don't get stuck thinking that because you are on a budget, you couldn't possibly afford to eat paleo. You definitely can, and it doesn't have to be perfect. If you can't eat everything organic, that's OK; you do the best with what you have. Small steps and small changes are what make lasting lifelong changes, so don't let your budget get in the way of changing the way you eat!

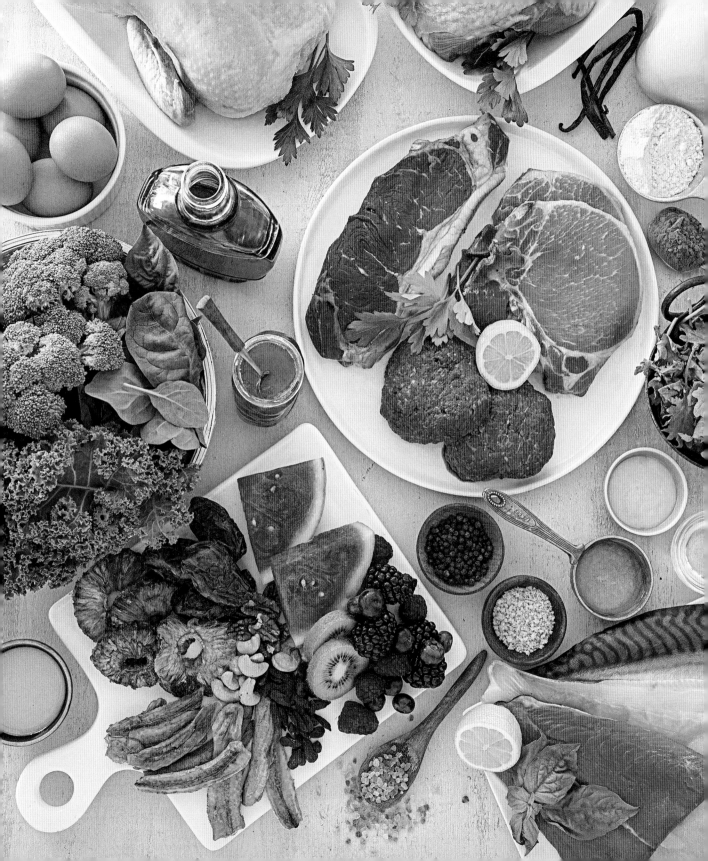

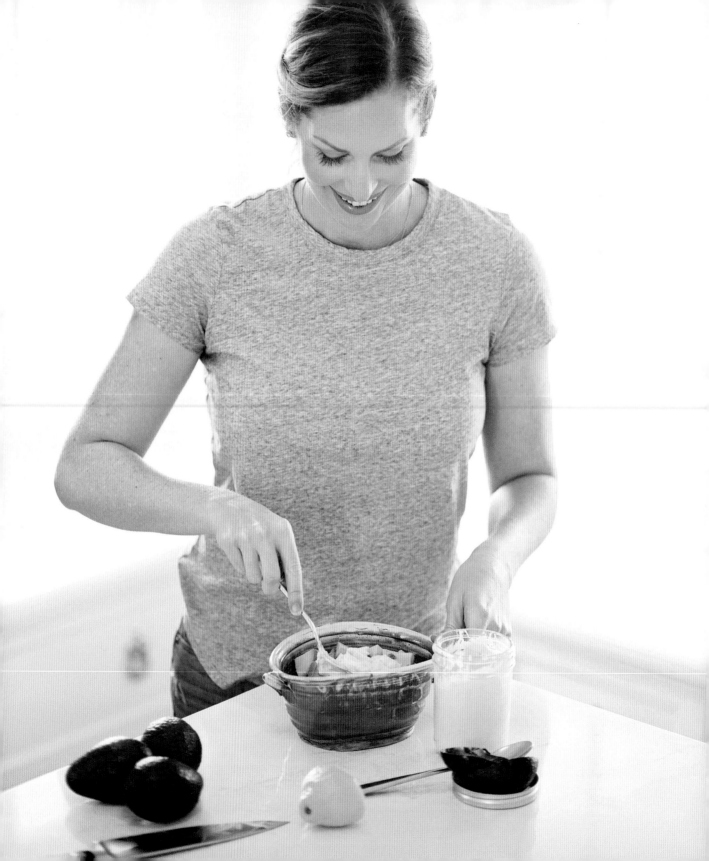

five

THE 30-DAY
THYROID RESET
RECIPES

What follows are some of my favorite recipes for a thyroid reset. You'll find delicious options for breakfast, lunch, and dinner, plus homemade staples you'll want to have on hand to avoid store-bought condiments. The Meal Plan on page 178 offers suggested recipes for the 30 days followed by a set of week-by-week shopping lists to make this reset as easy and stress-free as possible.

STAPLES

These are the basic recipes you should have on hand. They are simple to make and are used in many of the other recipes in this book.

HOMEMADE CHICKEN BONE BROTH

Chances are you have heard about all of the wonderful health benefits of bone broth, and its ability to support gut health is impressive. Bone broth is something that I recommend my patients include as part of their regular diet, and believe it or not it's actually really simple to make! You can simply add just a handful of the following ingredients to a slow cooker and let it work its magic. You will be left with a nourishing and delicious broth to use for the base of your favorite soup.

MAKES 12 CUPS (2.8 L)

1 chicken carcass

12 cups (2.8 L) filtered water

2 tbsp (30 ml) apple cider vinegar

2 ribs celery

2 large carrots, chopped

1 yellow onion, quartered

Herbs of choice

Start by adding the bones, filtered water, and apple cider vinegar to a large slow cooker.

Add the remaining ingredients. Cook on low for 8 to 10 hours.

Add more water if needed to make sure the bones and vegetables are covered throughout the entire cooking time.

Strain the broth through a fine-mesh strainer into glass jars and discard the bones and vegetables.

Let cool and then refrigerate. You can also freeze leftovers.

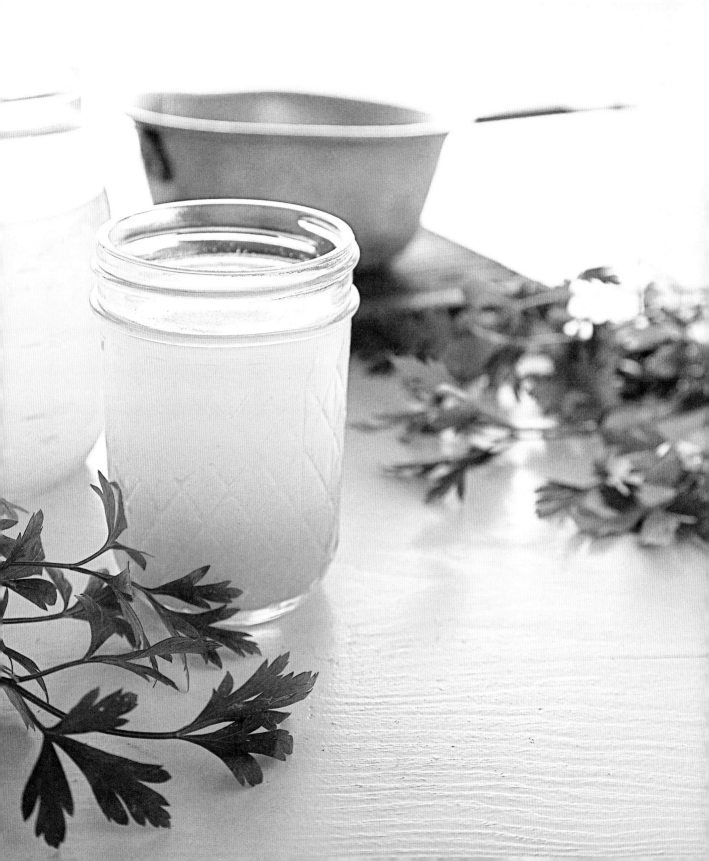

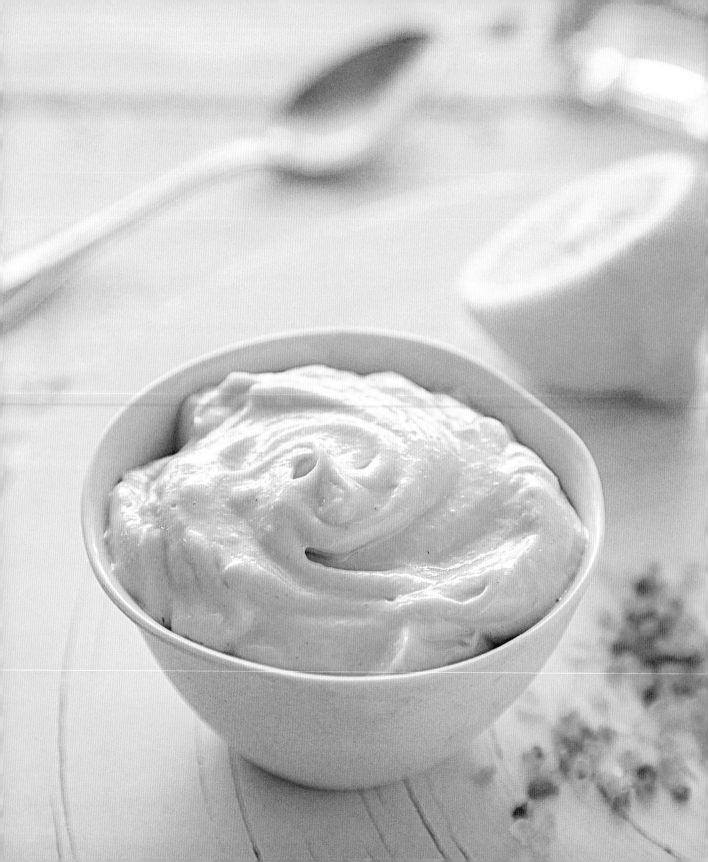

HOMEMADE PALEO-STYLE MAYONNAISE

Many of my patients are surprised to learn that they can still eat mayonnaise during the thyroid reset, but the trick here is to make your own. Making your own mayonnaise is super simple, only requires a handful of ingredients, and is absolutely delicious. My favorite way to enjoy this homemade mayo is slathered on cassava wraps (page 106).

MAKES 1 CUP (240 ML)

1 cup (240 ml) extra light tasting olive oil

1 egg

Juice of ½ lemon

1 tbsp (15 ml) sugar-free Dijon mustard (I use Annie's Organic)

½ tsp pink Himalayan sea salt

Add the olive oil to a canning-style jar and then add the egg, lemon juice, mustard, and salt.

Next, place an immersion blender into the canning jar. Turn it on low, blending until a mayonnaise consistency forms.

Store in the refrigerator.

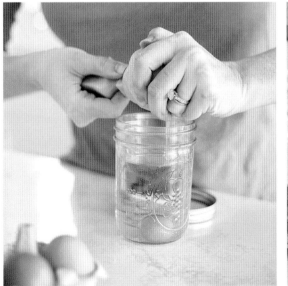
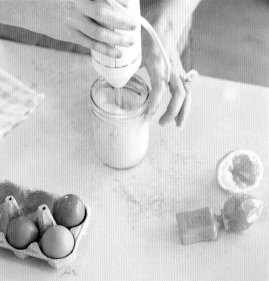

ROSEMARY AIOLI

This aioli pairs wonderfully with meat-based dishes and has the perfect combination of flavors. The rosemary really brings out the lemon juice and there is just a subtle hint of garlic. One of my favorite ways to use this sauce is in place of red sauce served over meatballs.

MAKES 1 CUP (240 ML)

1 cup (240 ml) Homemade Paleo-Style Mayonnaise (page 101)

2 tbsp (3 g) chopped rosemary

2 cloves garlic, flattened and minced

Juice of ½ lemon

Simply add the mayonnaise, chopped rosemary, and garlic to a mixing bowl and stir to combine.

Squeeze in the lemon juice and stir again.

Store in the fridge until ready to use.

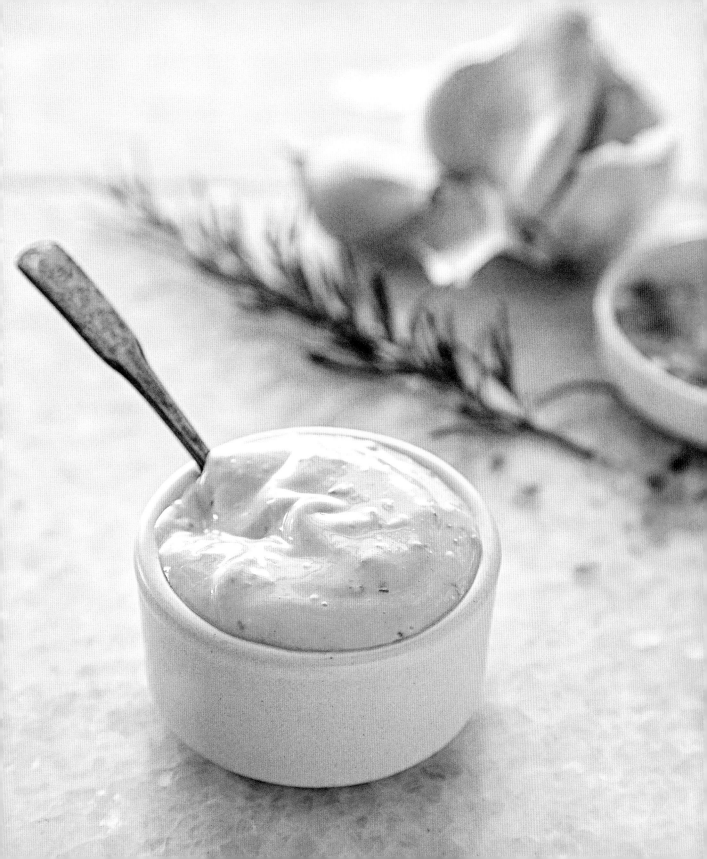

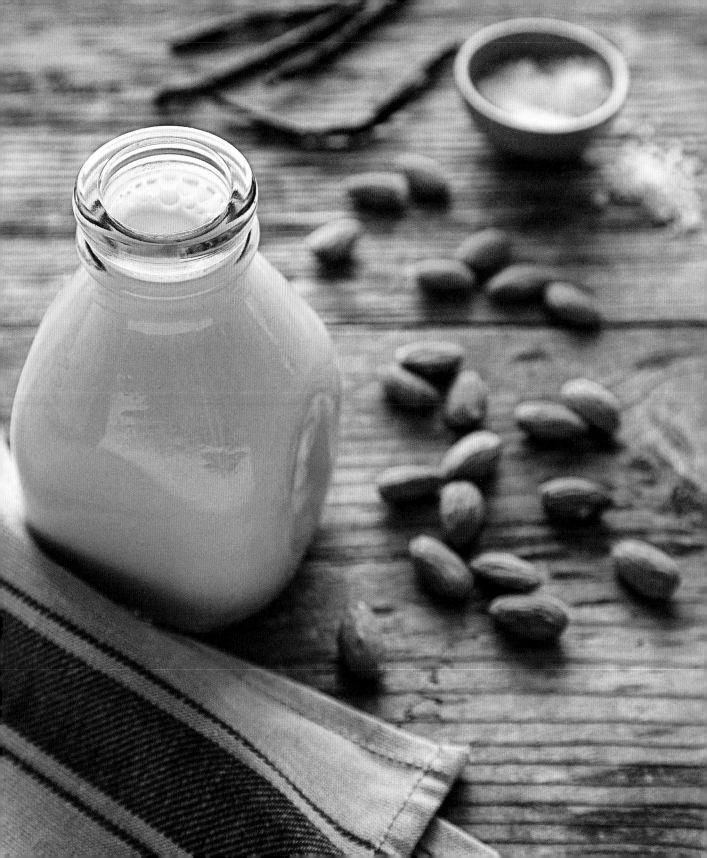

HOMEMADE VANILLA ALMOND MILK

You will find almond milk in many of the smoothie recipes throughout the 30-Day Thyroid Reset, and this homemade almond milk will blow any store-bought option out of the water. Not only does it taste amazing, but it is so much better for you. Instead of using the store-bought almond milk, make your own with just a handful of wholesome ingredients. You will be left with a creamy and decadent milk to use as the base for your smoothies.

MAKES 3 CUPS (720 ML)

1 cup (150 g) soaked raw almonds (soak the almonds overnight in filtered water and then drain and rinse well before using)

3 cups (720 ml) filtered water

Pinch of sea salt

1 tbsp (5 g) scraped vanilla bean

Simply add the soaked and rinsed almonds to a high-speed blender with the filtered water and salt and blend for 45 to 60 seconds.

Add the scraped vanilla beans and blend for another 30 seconds.

Strain the milk through a nut milk bag into a glass jar.

Store in the refrigerator for up to 2 days.

CASSAVA TORTILLAS

These are one of my all-time favorite base recipes to use with chicken or egg salad or just about any recipe that would call for traditional wheat-based wraps. They only take a couple of minutes to make, and they add in a healthy dose of carbohydrates, which is important for thyroid patients. Pair these wraps with some homemade mayonnaise, and you wouldn't even guess these wraps were gluten-free.

MAKES 10 TO 14 TORTILLAS

2½ cups (373 g) cassava flour

1 tsp sea salt

7 tbsp (105 ml) olive oil

1 to 2 cups (240 to 480 ml) water

Start by adding the flour and salt to a large mixing bowl and stir.

Add in the olive oil and water and stir well to form a dough that sticks together.

Next, preheat a large griddle to 300°F (149°C).

Form the dough into 10 to 14 small rounds and place each one between parchment paper. Flatten to form a tortilla shape.

Next, add the dough to the griddle and cook for about 3 minutes on each side.

Store by placing each cooked tortilla between 2 pieces of parchment paper.

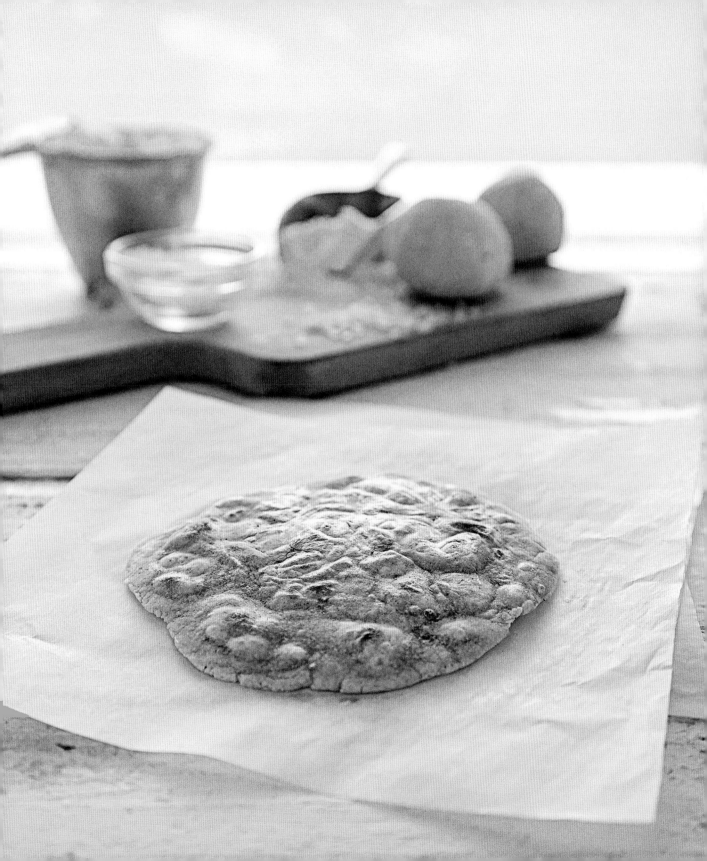

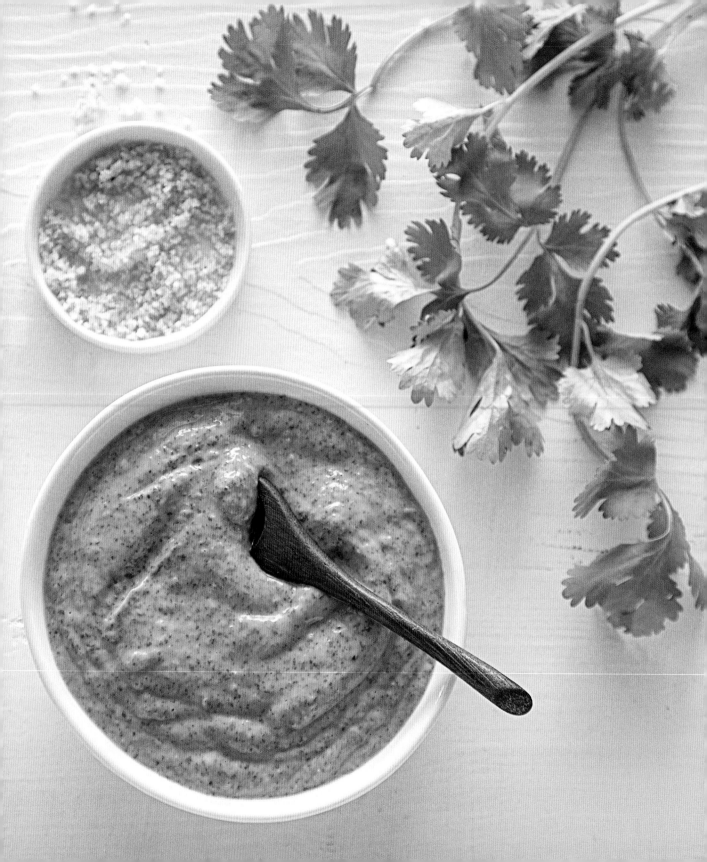

GREEN SAUCE

This green sauce is absolutely delicious and packed full of flavor. I love this sauce with tacos as it brings out the flavors from the seasoning. It provides a nice dose of nutritional value from the fiber and healthy fats from the avocados to the naturally detoxifying properties from the cilantro and lemon juice. The best part about this recipe is that all you need to do is add all the ingredients to a food processor and hit blend.

MAKES 1 CUP (240 ML)

1 avocado, peeled and pitted

1 bunch of cilantro, stems removed

1 to 2 cloves garlic, peeled

Juice of ½ lemon

½ to ¾ tsp salt

¾ cup (180 ml) extra light tasting olive oil

Simply place the avocado, cilantro, garlic, lemon juice, and salt in a food processor.

Start to pour in the olive oil as you are processing the other ingredients. You can add more olive oil if needed depending on how thick you like the sauce.

BREAKFASTS

In this section, you will find well-balanced recipes to get your day off on the right foot. Each recipe is designed to fuel your body with the nutrients it needs to help keep your blood sugar levels balanced and your energy levels high, with no sacrifice in flavor. I have included some of my go-to breakfast recipes, favorite smoothies, and savory dishes.

EGG MUFFINS

(Have the Breakfast Pork Patties, page 126, instead if following Option 2.)

These egg muffins are perfect for kids, as they taste delicious and sneak in some vegetables. You can easily make these muffins ahead of time and freeze them. Just pop however many you want for breakfast out of the freezer the night before to defrost in the fridge, then reheat and grab and go in the morning.

MAKES 12 MUFFINS

4 strips thick cut nitrate-free organic bacon

2 green onions, finely chopped (whites and greens)

½ small red onion, finely chopped

1 clove garlic, minced

2 cups (60 g) fresh spinach, finely chopped

½ tsp sea salt, divided

12 organic pasture-raised eggs

1 handful of fresh cilantro, chopped

Homemade Paleo-Style Mayonnaise (page 101) or Rosemary Aioli (page 102) for serving (optional)

Preheat the oven to 350°F (177°C) and line a 12-cup muffin tray with liners.

Next, heat a medium skillet over medium heat. Cut the bacon into pieces and brown. With a slotted spoon, remove the bacon and keep the bacon fat in the pan.

Add the green onion, red onion, and garlic to the pan and sauté over medium heat for 6 minutes and then add the spinach and sauté for an additional 2 minutes. Season with ¼ teaspoon of the salt.

Next, whisk the eggs in a large mixing bowl and add the cilantro and remaining ¼ teaspoon salt. Add the sautéed vegetables and whisk again. Pour the mixture into the muffin liners, filling each cup half full.

Bake for 20 to 25 minutes or until a toothpick inserted into the center comes out clean. Let cool. Serve with mayonnaise or aioli if desired.

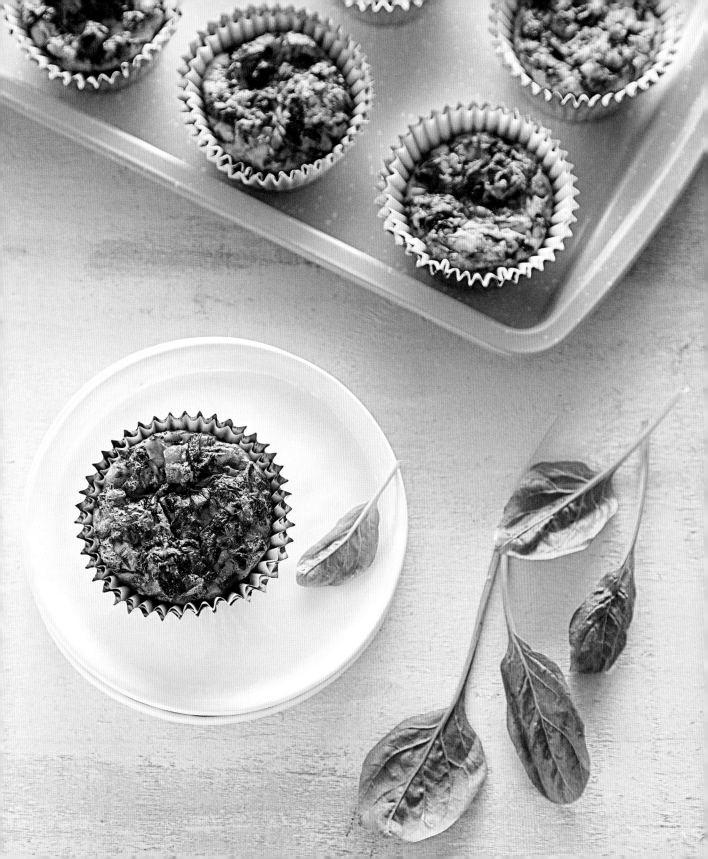

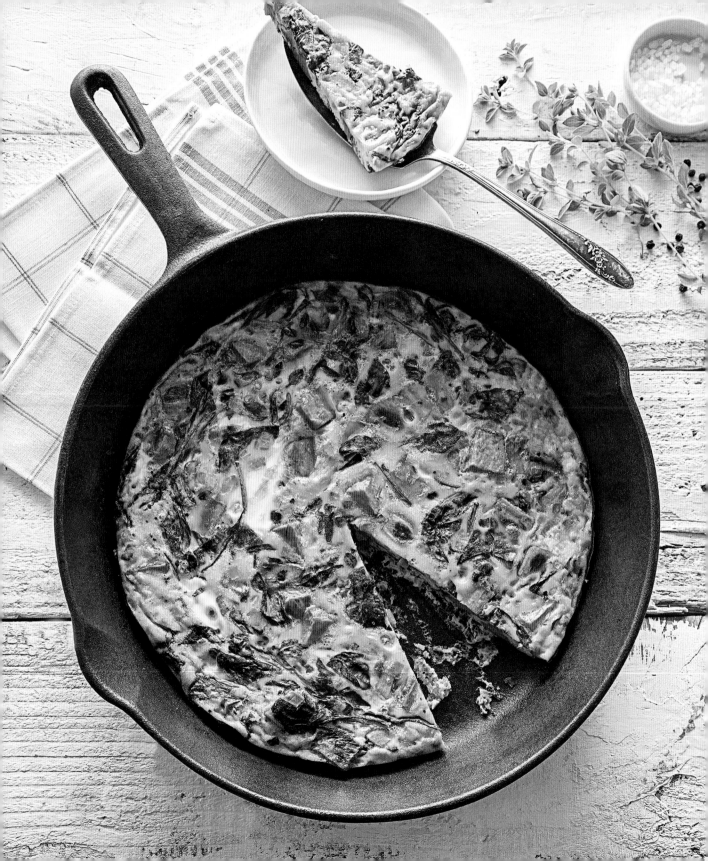

SWEET POTATO EGG FRITTATA

(Have the Coconut Kefir Parfait, page 125, instead if following Option 2.)

If you're looking for a healthy way to impress your guests while you are following the 30-Day Thyroid Reset, I highly recommend this recipe. This sweet potato frittata makes for the perfect healthy brunch option and is always a hit. With the delicious combination of garlic, onion, and herbs, this frittata can't go wrong. You can also make this ahead of time as an easy grab-and-go breakfast that you can store in the fridge or freeze for later use.

SERVES 6

1 sweet potato, peeled and cubed

2 tbsp (30 g) coconut oil, divided

⅜ tsp Himalayan pink sea salt, divided

1 yellow onion, chopped

2 cloves garlic, chopped

1 handful fresh spinach

1 tbsp (3 g) fresh oregano or 1 tsp dried

8 organic pasture-raised eggs

¼ tsp ground black pepper

Start by preheating the oven to 400°F (204°C) and placing the peeled and cubed sweet potato on a baking sheet lined with parchment paper. Coat the potatoes with 1 tablespoon (15 g) of the oil and ⅛ teaspoon of the salt. Cook for 20 minutes, then remove.

Turn the oven down to 350°F (177°C).

Next, preheat a cast-iron skillet over medium heat. Add the remaining 1 tablespoon (15 g) of oil and the onion and cook for 15 minutes.

Add the garlic and cook for 3 minutes, then add the spinach and the oregano and cook for an additional 2 to 3 minutes.

In a large bowl, beat the eggs, then add the sautéed onion mixture and the remaining ½ teaspoon of salt to combine all ingredients.

Next, add the egg mixture back to the skillet, and turn off the heat. Stir just until the egg mixture combines.

Place in the oven and bake for 20 minutes, or until the eggs are cooked through.

Slice into 6 pieces for serving.

Store any leftovers in the fridge.

NOTE: See note about goitrogens on page 85.

CREAMY BERRY SMOOTHIE

If you love berries as much as I do, then you are going to love this smoothie recipe. This smoothie has a subtle vanilla flavor from the homemade almond milk with hints of coconut from the coconut butter. Not only does this smoothie taste amazing, but it's also incredibly healthy for you, as it's balanced with protein from the almond milk, carbohydrates from the fruit, and healthy fat from the coconut butter. If you are in a rush to get out the door to work, this would be a great on-the-go breakfast option. Use coconut milk if you are following Option 2.

SERVES 1

1 cup (240 ml) Homemade Vanilla Almond Milk (page 105)

½ frozen banana

¼ cup (35 g) frozen blueberries

¾ cup (112 g) frozen strawberries

1 tbsp (15 ml) coconut butter

1 serving of paleo protein powder

Start by adding the almond milk to the blender followed by the frozen banana, berries, coconut butter, and protein powder.

Blend until smooth.

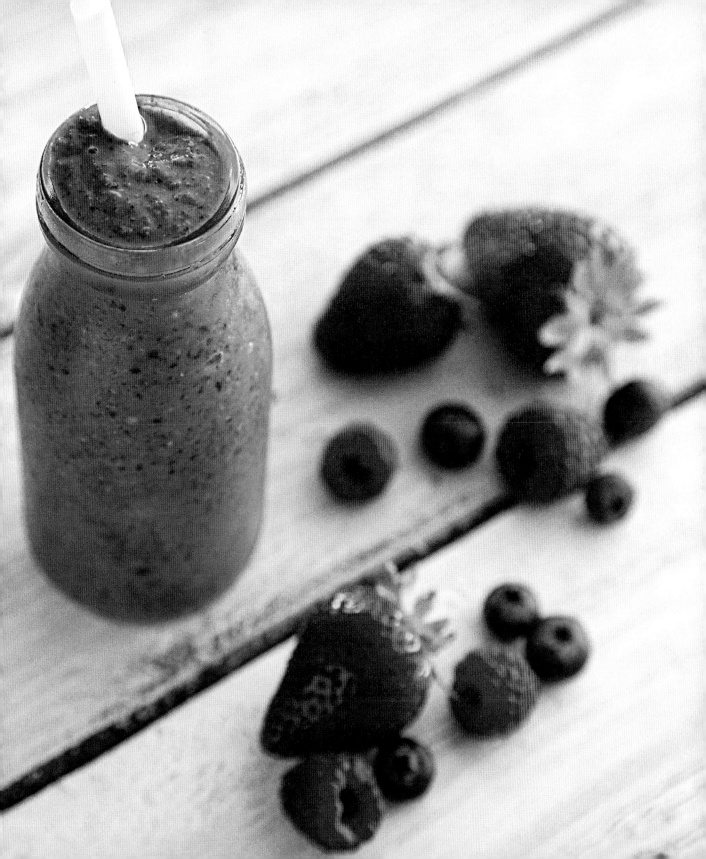

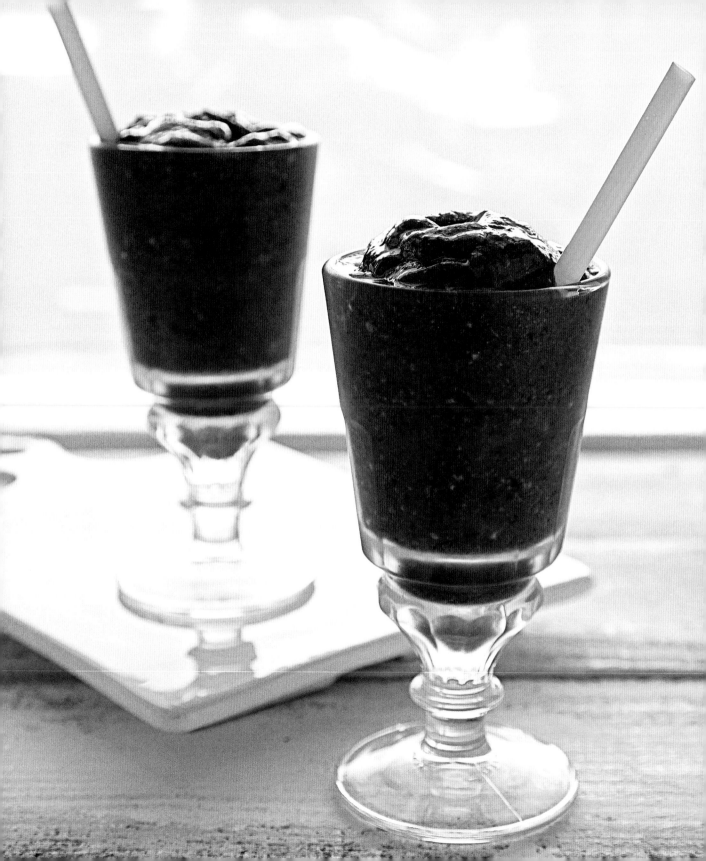

BERRY ANTIOXIDANT SMOOTHIE

Antioxidants are an important part of the thyroid reset because they can help better control inflammation in the body. When you are suffering from an autoimmune condition your body is already in an inflammatory state, so adding some antioxidant-rich foods such as berries can do your body a ton of good! This smoothie is also super easy to make and packs in a high dose of nutrition in just one single meal with little to no prep or cleanup time. It's the perfect option for those who are running out the door to work or school in the morning and just need something that they can quickly throw together that will help support their overall health. Use coconut milk if you are following Option 2.

SERVES 1

1 cup (240 ml) Homemade Vanilla Almond Milk (page 85)

½ plantain

¾ cup (112 g) frozen mixed berries (preferably organic)

1 tbsp (9 g) chia seeds

1 tbsp (15 ml) unsweetened coconut butter

1 serving of paleo protein powder

Start by adding the almond milk to the blender followed by the plantain, frozen mixed berries, chia seeds, coconut butter, and protein powder.

Blend until smooth.

CREAMY AVOCADO MINT SMOOTHIE

If you like mint chocolate chip milkshakes, this smoothie is for you. This creamy avocado smoothie is the perfect refreshing yet nourishing way to start your morning. The avocado provides your body with a healthy serving of fat and fiber while the flaxseeds add a nice dose of plant-based omega-3 fatty acids. Try this smoothie on a hot day or when you are looking for something quick yet satisfying before your hectic schedule begins. Use coconut milk if following Option 2.

SERVES 1

1 cup (240 ml) Homemade Vanilla Almond Milk (page 85)

1 frozen banana

½ avocado, pitted and peeled

2 tbsp (13 g) ground flaxseeds

1 handful of fresh spinach

3 fresh mint leaves

1 serving of paleo protein powder

Start by adding the almond milk to the blender followed by the banana, avocado, flaxseeds, spinach, mint leaves, and the protein powder.

Blend until smooth.

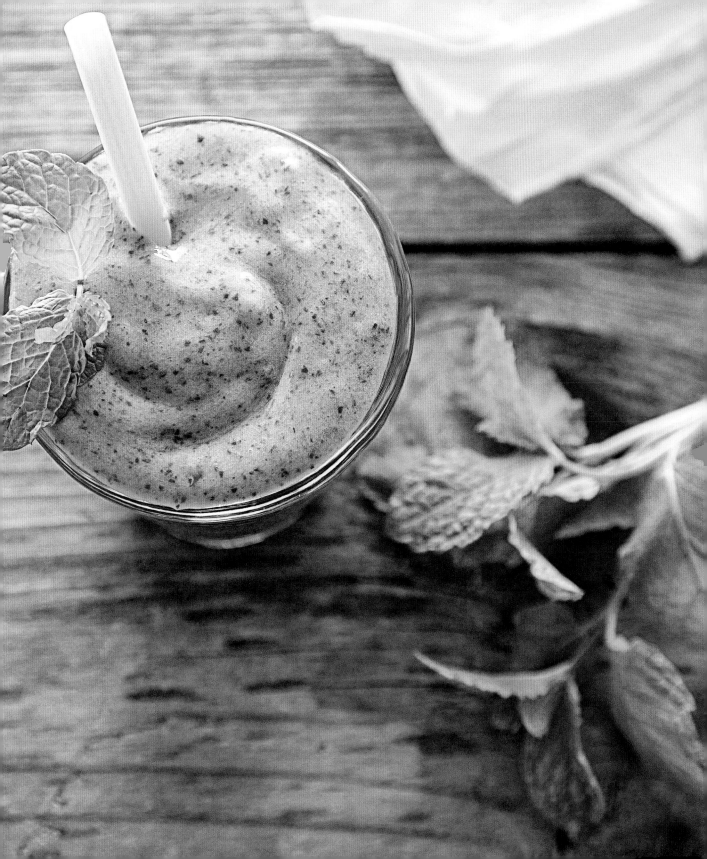

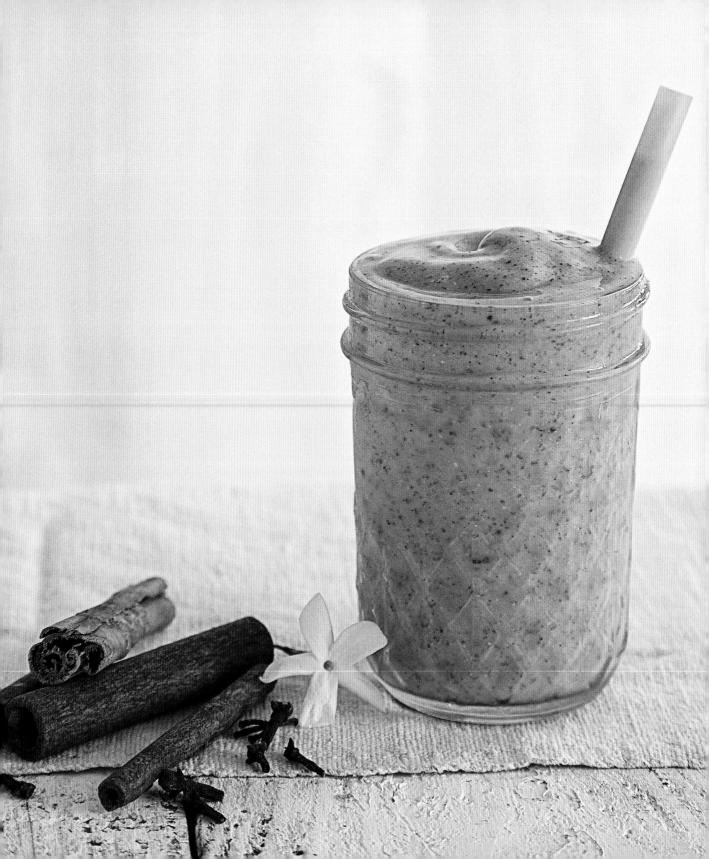

VANILLA CHAI SMOOTHIE

I don't know about you, but I love vanilla! The pure vanilla bean in this smoothie truly brings out all of the other delicious flavors from the spices. This smoothie has the perfect balance of sweet yet savory and is an excellent way to start your morning. Pack in a healthy dose of omega-3 fatty acids from the chia seeds and some potassium and fiber from the banana, and you have yourself a nutritious, easy-to-make breakfast. Use coconut milk if following Option 2.

SERVES: 1

1 cup (240 ml) Homemade Vanilla Almond Milk (page 85)

1 frozen banana

½ tsp ground cinnamon

¼ tsp ground ginger

¼ tsp ground cloves

1 tsp pure vanilla bean seeds

1 tbsp (9 g) chia seeds

1 serving of paleo protein powder

Start by adding the almond milk to the blender followed by the banana, cinnamon, ginger, cloves, vanilla bean seeds, chia seeds, and protein powder.

Blend until smooth.

BREAKFAST SAUSAGE AND EGGS

Sausage and eggs is a classic breakfast option, but it isn't always the healthiest choice. This is why I created a healthy spinoff that includes lots of fresh herbs and spices and veggies to get your day started off on the right foot. A nice dose of protein from the sausage and eggs will keep you feeling full until lunchtime. I love this recipe on the weekends when I have a little more time to prep breakfast, and the whole family loves this recipe. Eliminate eggs and bell pepper if following Option 2.

SERVES 1

Coconut oil for cooking

1 tbsp (10 g) chopped white onion

1 clove garlic, chopped

¼ green bell pepper, diced

1 organic nitrate-free chicken sausage, diced (about 4 oz, or 112 g)

Chili powder (to taste)

2 organic pasture-raised eggs

Sea salt and pepper to taste

Start by preheating a large skillet over medium heat with the coconut oil.

Add the onions to the skillet and sauté until caramelized, about 5 minutes.

Add the garlic, green pepper, and sausage and cook for another 5 to 7 minutes, or until the sausage is cooked and all of the vegetable are soft.

Season with the chili powder.

Crack the eggs into a separate pan with additional coconut oil and cook to your liking. An over-easy egg works well here.

Serve the sausage mixture with the cooked eggs.

Season the eggs with sea salt and pepper if desired.

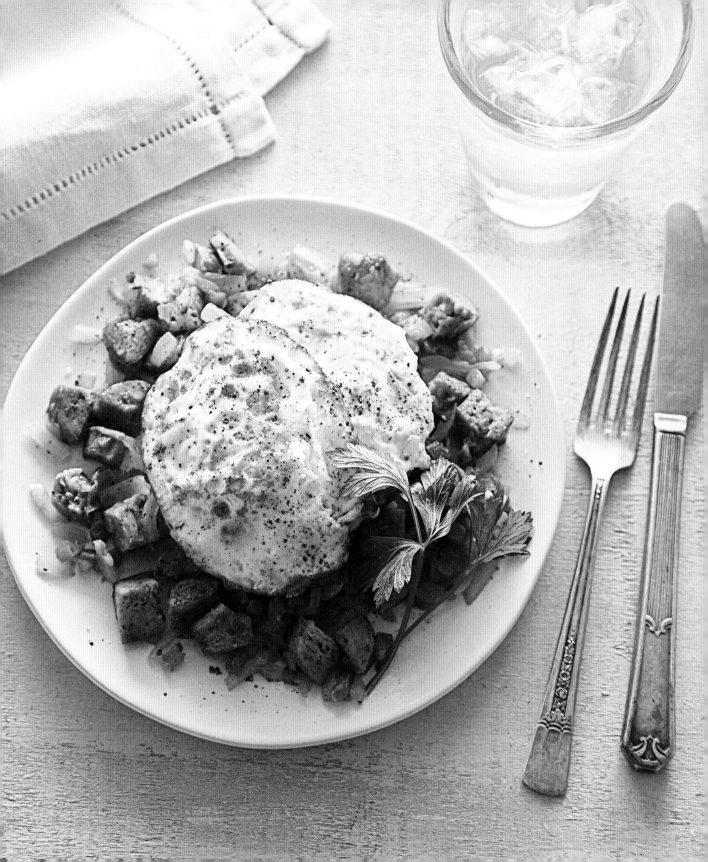

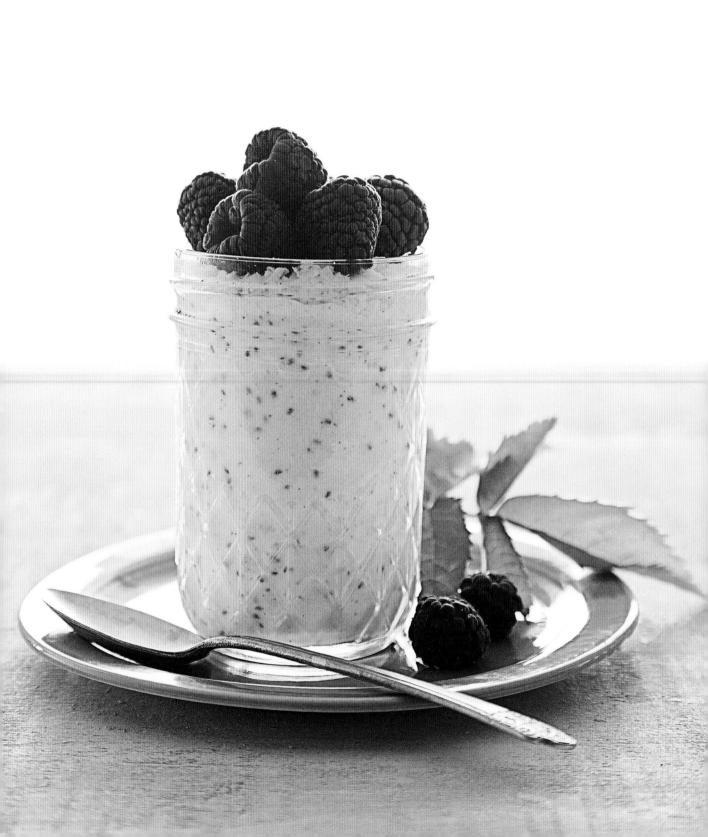

COCONUT KEFIR PARFAIT

Coconut and kefir are the perfect pair to help support gut health. This is one of my go-to breakfast recipes when I am in need of a little digestive boost. The coconut kefir is super creamy and the added superfoods make this an anti-inflammatory yet super filling breakfast that takes little to no time to throw together. You can even make this the night before in a Mason-style jar and keep it in the fridge to grab before you head out the door in the morning.

SERVES 4

4 cups (960 ml) coconut kefir

2 tsp (10 g) cinnamon

4 tbsp (36 g) chia seeds

4 tbsp (24 g) shredded unsweetened coconut

1 cup (123 g) raspberries

Start by adding the coconut kefir to 4 canning jars or bowls, and then add the cinnamon and chia seeds. Stir to combine.

Top with the shredded coconut and raspberries.

PORK PATTIES

This recipe is a great way to start your day because it gives you a nice energizing protein boost. If you enjoy a more savory breakfast, you will love this recipe. The caramelized shallots pair perfectly with the Swiss chard, giving it a savory taste, so you will actually enjoy getting some greens in for breakfast!

SERVES 4

2 tbsp (30 ml) coconut oil, divided

1 lb (454 g) organic ground pork

½ tsp garlic powder

½ tsp onion powder

1 tsp dried parsley

½ tsp salt

2 shallots, sliced

1 bunch Swiss chard, chopped

Start by preheating a medium skillet over medium heat with 1 tablespoon (15 ml) of the coconut oil. Add the ground pork to a mixing bowl with the spices and salt. Form into 4 patties. Add the patties to the skillet.

While the patties are cooking, add the sliced shallots to another skillet with the remaining 1 tablespoon (15 ml) of coconut oil. Cook until caramelized. This should take about 5 minutes.

Add the Swiss chard and cook for another 10 minutes, until soft.

When the patties are browned, remove from the heat and serve on top of the bed of the caramelized chard mix. Serve with a side of fried plantains.

FRIED PLANTAINS

½ cup (120 ml) coconut oil

2 green plantains, sliced into ¼" (6-mm) circles

½ tsp garlic powder

¼ tsp salt

Heat a large skillet with the coconut oil over medium heat. Add the plantains, sprinkle evenly with the garlic and salt, and cook on each side until lightly brown, about 5 minutes per side.

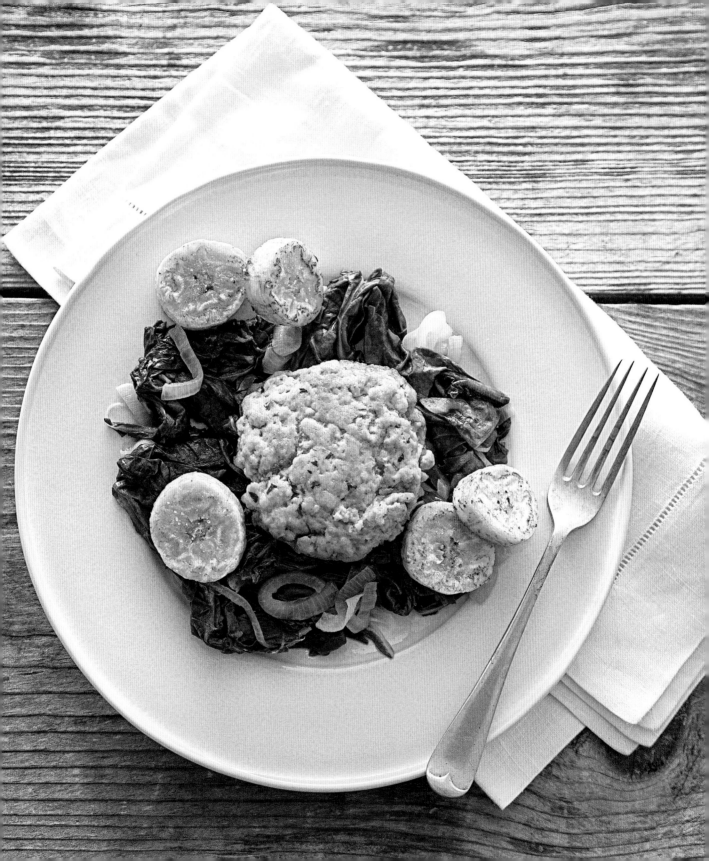

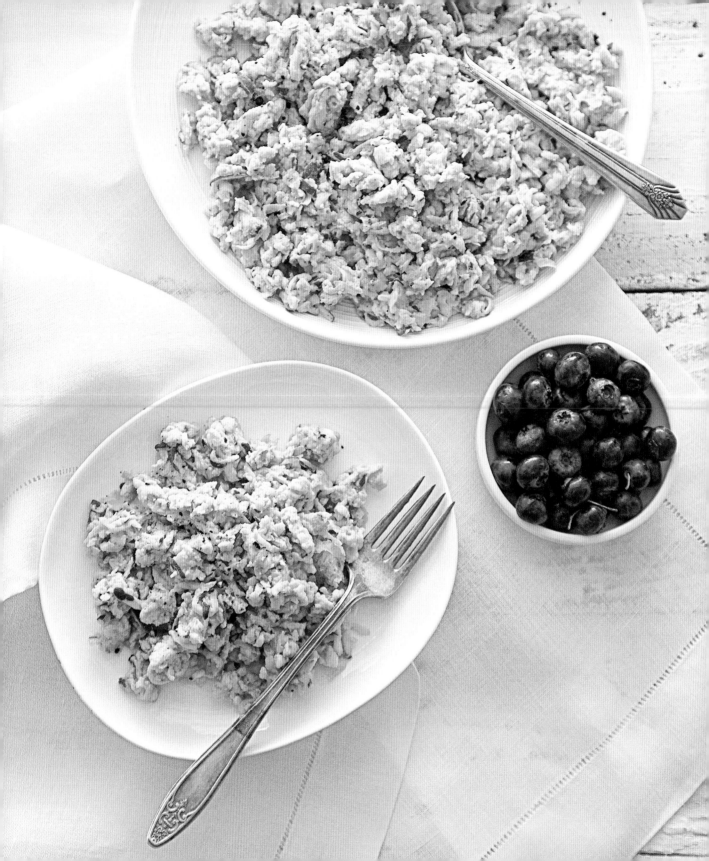

ZUCCHINI AND CARAMELIZED ONION SCRAMBLE

This recipe gives the traditional scrambled eggs a new spin. Eggs are a staple in my diet, but sometimes plain old scrambled or hard-boiled eggs get boring. This recipe adds some flavor and nutritional value from the veggies. What better way to get your day started than with a rich source of protein and a serving of veggies?

SERVES 4

8 organic pasture-raised eggs (or 1 lb [454 g] ground turkey breast if following Option 2)

Olive oil

1 large sweet Vidalia onion, chopped

1 zucchini, grated

Himalayan sea salt and pepper to taste

Fresh berries, for serving

Start by adding the eggs to a mixing bowl and whisk. (If using ground turkey, sauté it in a skillet until cooked through and then use in place of the eggs.)

Preheat a large skillet over medium heat with a drizzle of olive oil and add the onion. Sauté the onion until caramelized, about 10 minutes.

Add the zucchini and cook for an additional 5 minutes,

Add the eggs and season with salt and pepper. Cook until the eggs are firm.

Serve with some fresh berries.

LUNCHES

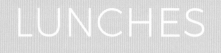

This section includes a balance of recipes that are ideal for those who need a quick grab-and-go lunch as well as dishes for when you have a bit of extra time to prep your midday meal. Lunch is a very important part of supporting thyroid health. It is crucial to fuel your body throughout the day and not let your blood sugar levels dip. For these recipes, I have included foods to help with just that and to help prevent that midafternoon energy crash. You will find a combination of soups, egg and chicken salads, and wraps.

SAUSAGE SOUP

This is one of my favorite soup recipes, as it's full of mild yet spicy flavor from the Italian sausage, and it's very simple to make. This is a great soup for the weekend and to have in the fridge for an easy weekday lunch or dinner.

SERVES 4

Olive oil

1 lb (454 g) ground organic nitrate-free mild Italian sausage

1 white onion, chopped

2 cloves garlic, minced

1 medium butternut squash, peeled and cut into cubes

1 carrot, chopped

1½ tsp (6 g) Italian seasoning

5 cups (1.2 L) Homemade Chicken Bone Broth (page 98)

½ cup (120 ml) full-fat coconut milk

3 cups (90 g) fresh spinach, chopped

1 handful freshly chopped basil

Salt and pepper to taste

Start by heating a large stockpot over medium heat with a splash of olive oil. Add the sausage and onion, and sauté until the sausage is thoroughly cooked through.

Next, add the garlic along with the cubed butternut squash, carrots, and seasoning and cook for another 3 to 5 minutes.

Add the bone broth and bring to a simmer. Simmer for about 20 minutes, or until the butternut squash is tender.

Add the coconut milk, spinach, basil, and salt and pepper and simmer for another couple of minutes.

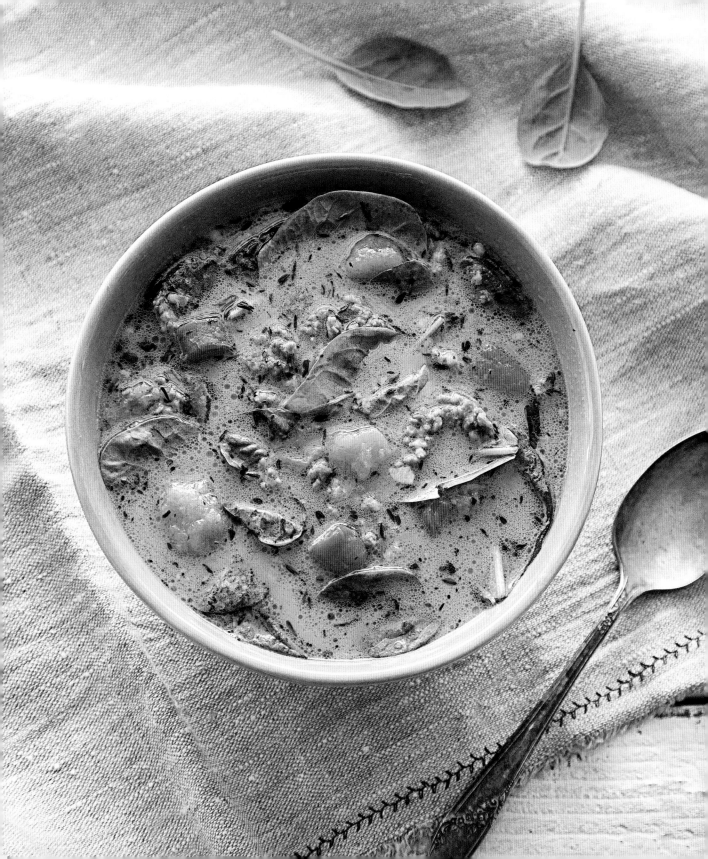

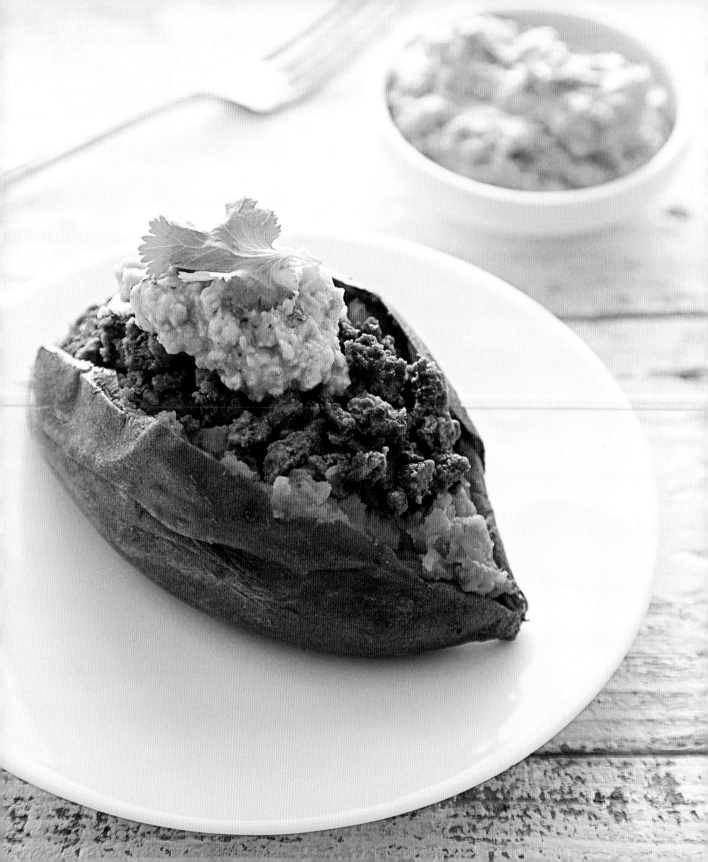

STUFFED SWEET POTATOES WITH ROASTED GARLIC GUACAMOLE

This is one of my favorite recipes and the addition of the roasted garlic guacamole brings all the flavors together perfectly. These stuffed sweet potatoes may not look like much, but they are super filling and loaded with nutrition. Between the grass-fed ground beef for a nice dose of protein, the sweet potatoes for complex carbohydrates and vitamin A, and the guacamole for healthy fat, these stuffed sweet potatoes are just about as balanced as you can get. You will find this recipe included in the lunch section of the thyroid reset, but feel free to enjoy them any time of day after the reset period is over. Believe it or not, they make an excellent breakfast option as well!

SERVES 4

4 large sweet potatoes

1 tbsp (15 ml) coconut oil

½ tsp garlic powder

½ tsp onion powder

¼ tsp salt

1 lb (454 g) organic grass-fed ground beef

1 batch Roasted Garlic Guacamole (page 134)

Start by preheating the oven to 400°F (204°C) and lining a baking sheet with parchment paper. Poke a few holes in the sweet potatoes and bake for 45 minutes to 1 hour, or until tender.

While the sweet potatoes are cooking, heat a medium skillet over medium heat with the coconut oil.

Mix the garlic and onion powders with the salt in a small dish.

Place the ground beef in the pan and top with the mixed seasoning. Cook the ground beef until browned.

Once the sweet potatoes are cooked, slice in half and mash down evenly. Fill the sweet potatoes with the cooked ground beef and top with the guacamole.

NOTE: Refer to the note about goitrogens on page 85.

ROASTED GARLIC GUACAMOLE

Olive oil

2 cloves garlic, skin on

3 ripe avocados, peeled and pitted

1 tbsp (10 g) finely chopped red onion

⅓ cup (5 g) fresh cilantro, stems removed and finely chopped

Juice of ½ to 1 lime

Sea salt to taste

Start by heating a small skillet over medium-low heat with a little drizzle of olive oil. Add the whole garlic cloves and cook for about 10 minutes, turning periodically. You will know they are done when they have black spots on the outside.

Allow the garlic cloves to cool and then remove the skin and add to a mixing bowl.

Mash the garlic and add the avocados, onion, cilantro, and lime juice. Mash together and then season with sea salt.

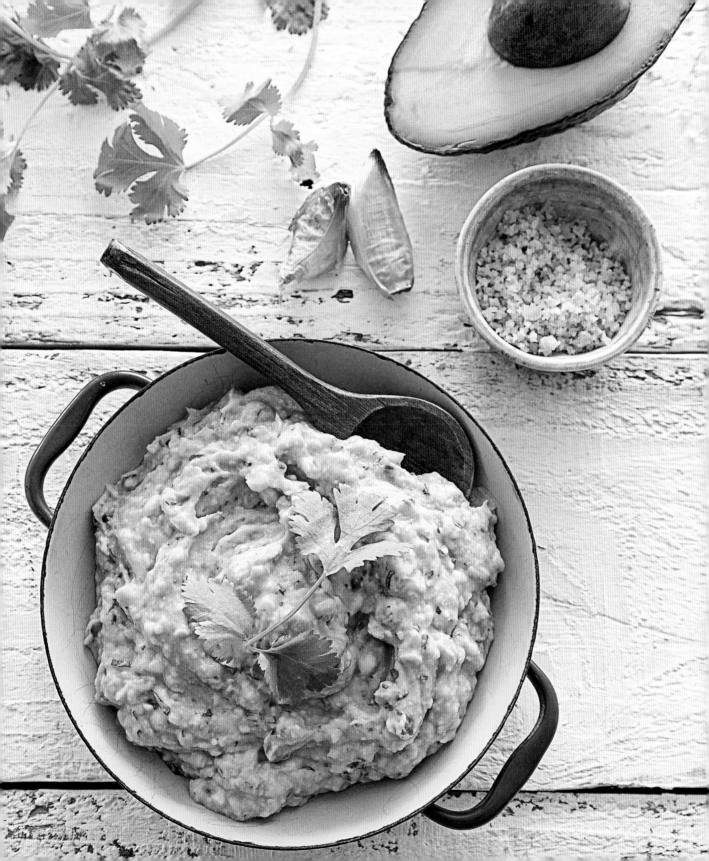

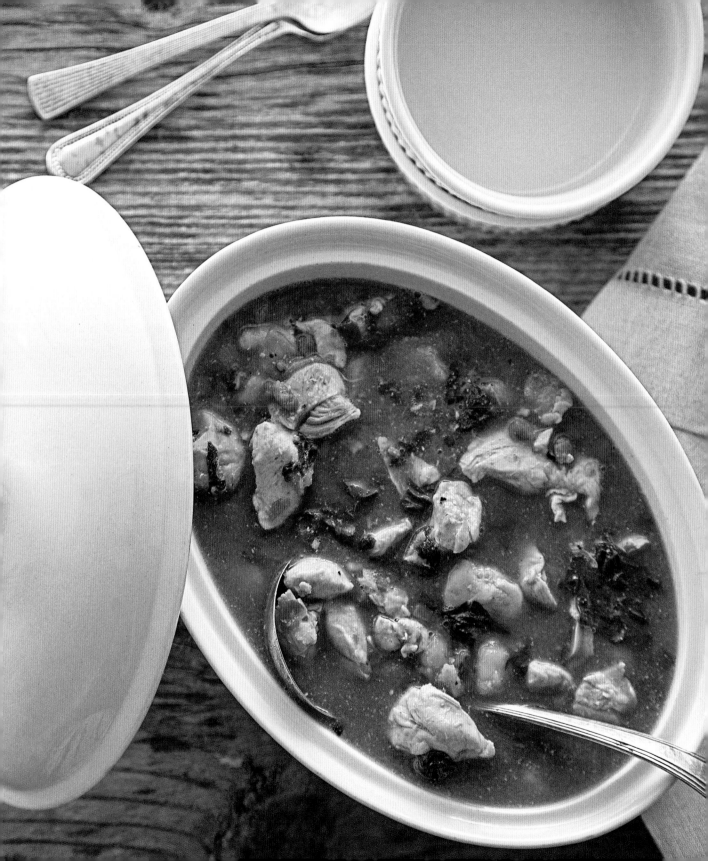

BONE BROTH CHICKEN SOUP

I don't know about you, but sometimes a good bowl of chicken noodle soup is what the body needs and this is something that I encourage my patients to enjoy regularly. The added bonus with this recipe is that it's made with homemade bone broth, which is excellent for anyone who suffers from digestive health issues, including leaky gut. Added into the soup are sweet potato cubes for healthy carbohydrates and the classic chicken and onion you would find in traditional chicken noodle soup. Even after the initial 30-day reset you may find yourself resorting back to this recipe when your body is in need of a gut health reboot or you are craving something nutrient dense on a cold fall or winter day.

SERVES 4

1 tbsp (15 ml) olive oil

1 yellow onion, chopped

4 chicken breasts, cubed

7 cups (1.7 L) Homemade Chicken Bone Broth (page 98)

2 carrots, chopped

1 medium white sweet potato, peeled and chopped (use a regular sweet potato if you cannot find a white sweet potato)

7 Swiss chard leaves, chopped

2 cloves garlic, chopped

Sea salt and pepper to taste

In a large stockpot, heat the olive oil over medium heat and add the onion. Cook for about 3 minutes.

Add the chicken and cook for an additional 5 minutes.

Add the broth, carrots, sweet potato, chard, and garlic to the stockpot and bring to a simmer.

Simmer for 25 to 30 minutes, or until the sweet potatoes are tender and the chicken is cooked through, adding more broth during the cooking time if needed.

Season with salt and pepper.

NOTE: Refer to the note about goitrogens on page 85.

HEALTHY EGG SALAD

If well-tolerated, eggs are something that I recommend my patients enjoy, as they contain essential vitamins and minerals to support overall health. They are also an excellent source of healthy fat and protein. This egg salad recipe is a healthy spin on the traditional egg salad. Instead of store-bought mayo, you use the homemade version and mashed avocado (optional) to add that creamy consistency with extra health benefits. If you choose to add fresh dill, it gives the salad a unique yet refreshing taste.

SERVES 4

8 hard-boiled eggs, cooled and peeled

½ cup (120 ml) Homemade Paleo-Style Mayonnaise (page 101)

2 tbsp (30 ml) spicy mustard or sugar-free Dijon mustard

2 tbsp (5 g) chopped fresh dill

1 avocado, peeled, pitted, and cubed (optional)

½ tsp sea salt

¼ tsp black pepper

Large lettuce leaves or Cassava Tortillas (page 106), for serving

Add the eggs to a large mixing bowl and mash together with the mayonnaise and mustard, and stir well to combine.

Add the dill and avocado, if using, and salt and pepper and stir again.

Serve with large lettuce leaves or cassava tortillas.

NOTE: Have Stuffed Sweet Potatoes (page 133) or Bone Broth Chicken Soup (page 98) instead if following Option 2.

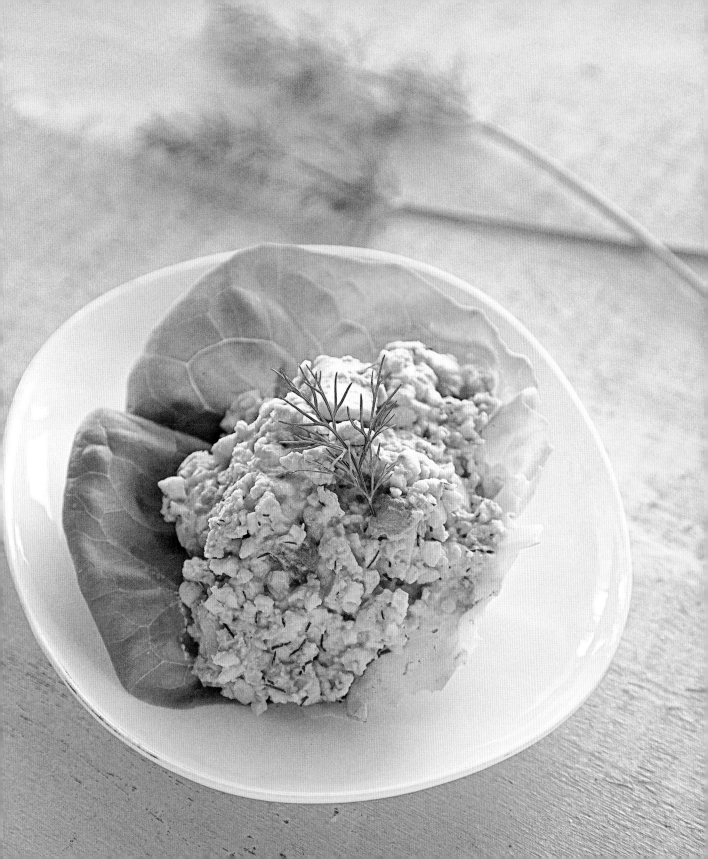

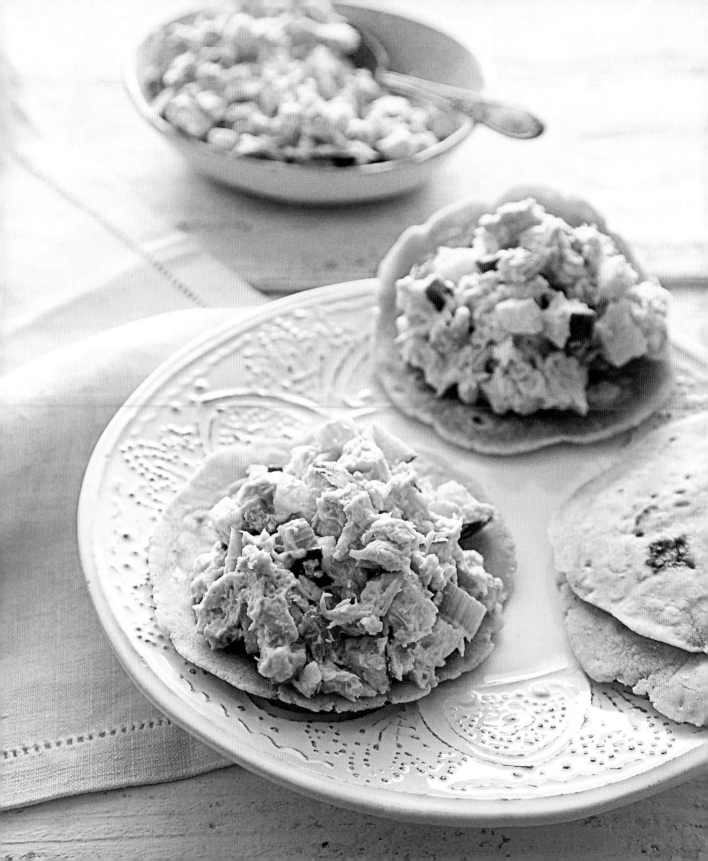

CHICKEN SALAD

Chicken salad is one of my go-to lunch options because it's simple to make and is one of my favorite recipes to pair with coconut or cassava wraps. You can easily make a large batch of this ahead of time to keep in the fridge to enjoy during the week. The coconut wraps are my favorite for this recipe.

SERVES 4

1 whole chicken

1 cup (240 ml) Homemade Chicken Bone Broth (page 98)

½ cup (120 ml) Homemade Paleo-Style Mayonnaise (page 101) (eliminate if following Option 2)

2 ribs celery, chopped

1 red apple, chopped

4 coconut wraps or Cassava Tortillas (page 106), for serving (optional)

Start by adding the chicken and the broth to a slow cooker and cook on high for 4 hours.

Once the chicken is cooked, remove the meat and cut it into small pieces. Mix the meat with the mayonnaise (unless following Option 2), celery, and red apple and stir well to combine.

Serve with coconut wraps or cassava tortillas if desired.

AVOCADO AND CHICKEN WRAP

Wraps are always an easy go-to lunch when you live a busy lifestyle. Instead of buying a wrap or sandwich for lunch, make this avocado and chicken wrap to save money and provide your body with the nutrition that it is craving. The chicken gives your body the protein it needs to repair and also helps to keep you feeling full. The avocado and sauerkraut support gut health with fiber and healthy probiotics. Slather on some homemade mayonnaise, and you have yourself the perfect wrap.

SERVES 1

2 organic bone-in chicken breasts

2 tbsp (30 ml) Homemade Paleo-Style Mayonnaise (page 101) (eliminate if following Option 2)

1 avocado, peeled, pitted, and cubed

Juice of ½ lemon

Salt and pepper to taste

Lettuce leaf, coconut wrap, or Cassava Tortilla (page 106), for serving

OPTIONAL TOPPINGS

Small yellow onion, sliced

Sauerkraut

Bake the chicken at 375°F (190°C) for 45 minutes, or until cooked through.

Remove the chicken from the bone and chop into small pieces. Mix well with the mayonnaise, avocado, and lemon juice. Season with salt and pepper.

Assemble the wrap by adding the chicken mixture to the center of the wrap and top with the sliced onion and sauerkraut if desired.

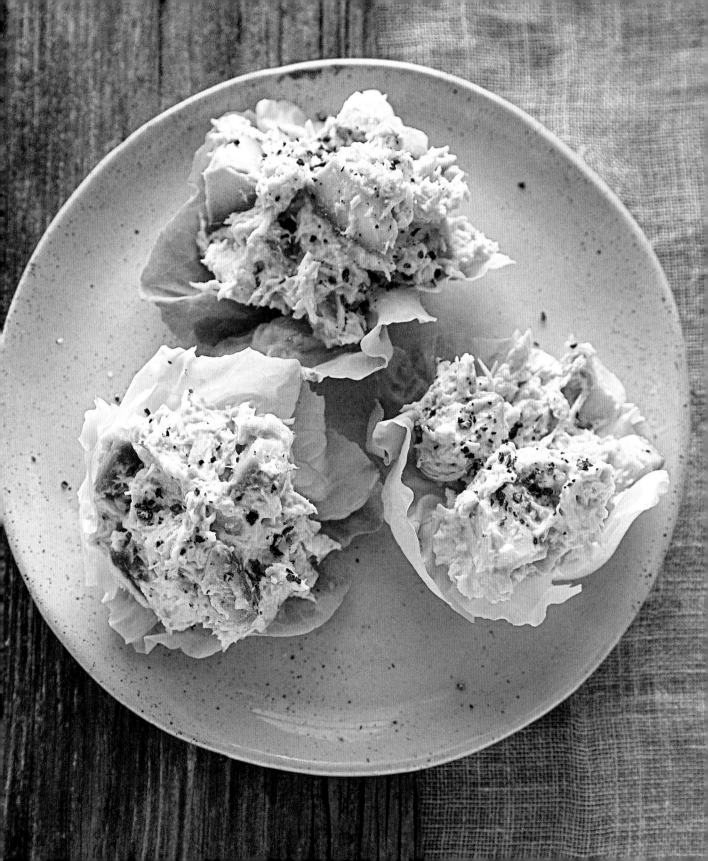

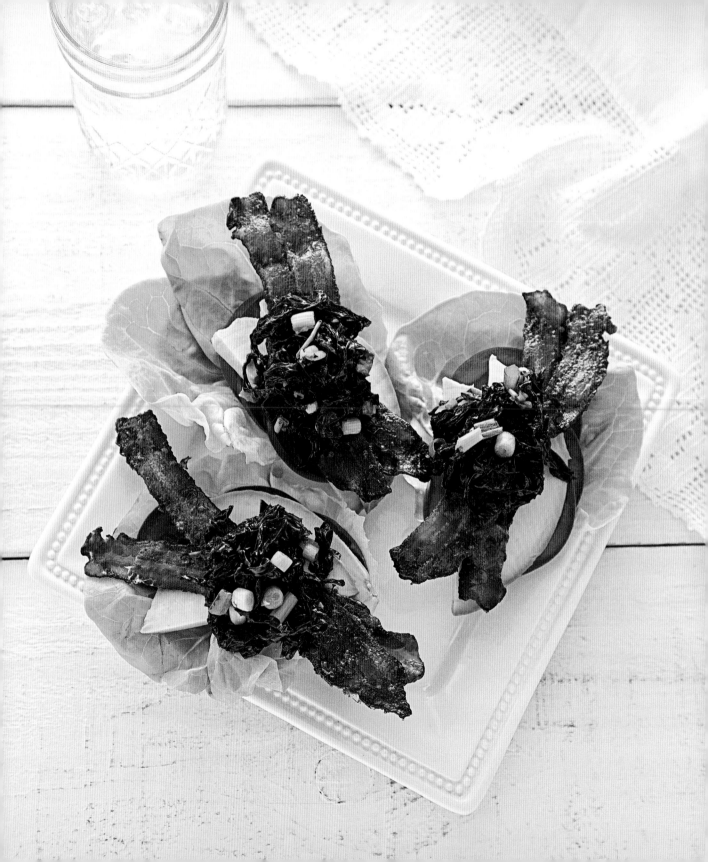

BLT WITH A SEAWEED SALAD

If you love bacon, lettuce, and tomato sandwiches, then you will love this recipe. Although not your traditional BLT, this recipe incorporates healthier ingredients with the same concept as a classic BLT. Paired with a seaweed salad, this lunch recipe has lots of thyroid-supporting benefits and quite a bit of fiber from the avocado to keep you feeling full until dinnertime.

SERVES 4

8 slices thick-cut nitrate-free organic bacon

½ cup (120 ml) Homemade Paleo-Style Mayonnaise (page 101)

8 large lettuce leaves or coconut wraps

2 avocados, peeled, pitted, and sliced

8 slices tomato (eliminate if following Option 2)

FOR THE SEAWEED SALAD

1 cup (80 g) dried wakame or dulse seaweed

2 tsp (10 g) freshly grated ginger

Juice of 2 lemons

4 green onions, finely chopped

Cook the bacon in a medium skillet over medium heat until desired crispiness.

Assemble the sandwich by spreading the mayo onto the lettuce leaves or wraps and topping it with the avocado, cooked bacon, and tomato (unless following Option 2).

Make the seaweed salad by mixing the seaweed, ginger, lemon juice, and green onion together in a mixing bowl and serve alongside the BLT.

NOTE: Have the Avocado Chicken Wrap (page 142) or the Chicken Salad (page 141) with the appropriate modifications instead if you are following Option 2.

WILD SALMON SALAD

I love adding salmon to my diet, and I often recommend that my patients try enjoying more omega-3-rich foods to help combat inflammation. This wild salmon salad is perfect for the warmer months, but you can truly enjoy it any time of the year. It's simple to make, high in protein and healthy fat, and one of my go-to options when I am looking to eat something on the lighter side.

SERVES 4

4 cups (80 g) fresh arugula

4 cups (120 g) fresh spinach

4 (6-oz [170-g]) cans wild-caught salmon, drained

½ cup (120 ml) Homemade Paleo-Style Mayonnaise (page 101) (use 2 tbsp [30 ml] extra virgin olive oil if following Option 2)

¼ tsp sea salt

⅛ tsp black pepper

1 cup (134 g) green olives, sliced

2 tomatoes, quartered (eliminate if following Option 2)

Olive oil, for drizzling or (optional)

Arrange the arugula and spinach on a serving plate.

Mix the salmon with the mayonnaise or oil and season with salt and pepper.

Add the salmon to the salad with the olives and tomato.

Drizzle with olive oil if desired.

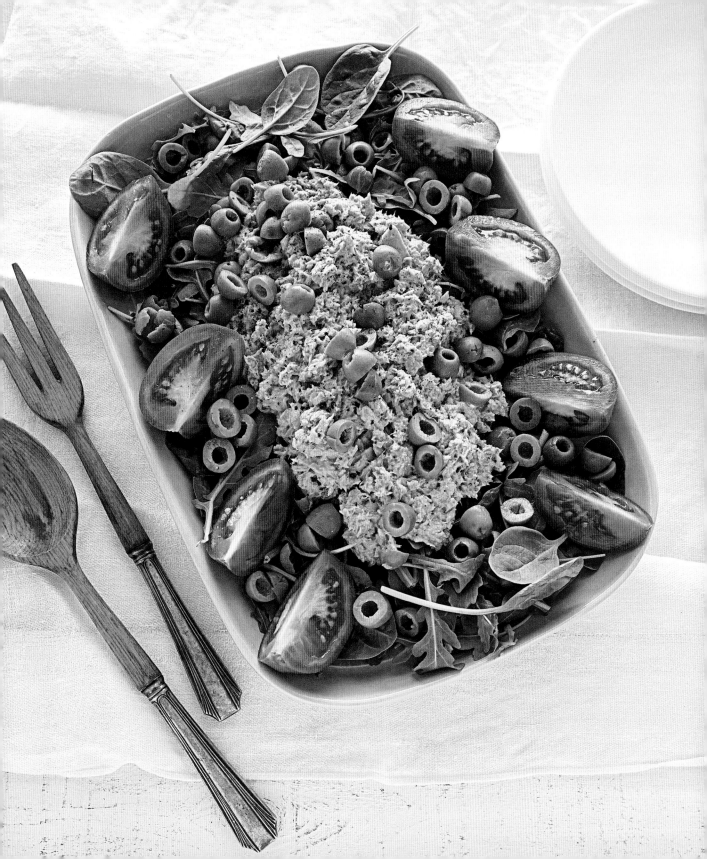

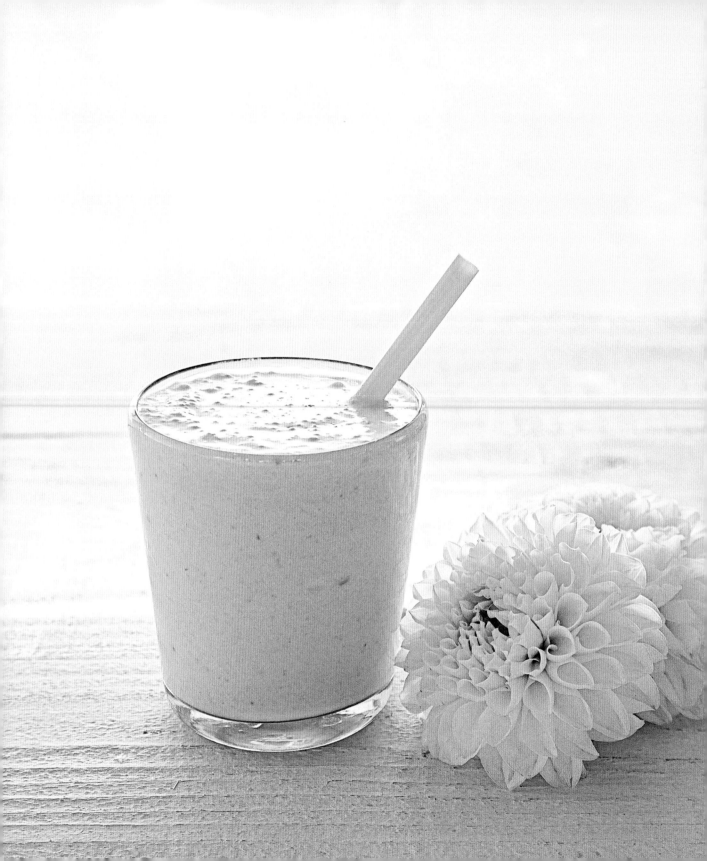

ON-THE-GO YOUNG COCONUT AND PEACH LUNCH SHAKE

On days where you just don't have time to prepare lunch, this on-the-go lunch shake is the perfect option. It balances fat and carbohydrates to keep you feeling full while also supporting a healthy digestive system. The combination of peaches and coconut is also out-of-this-world good. You may love this recipe so much that it becomes a staple part of your diet. I frequently find myself blending up this shake for a healthy snack when hunger pangs kick in. If you are following Option 2, omit the almond milk and substitute additional coconut milk.

SERVES 1

1 cup (240 ml) full-fat unsweetened coconut milk

½ cup (120 ml) Homemade Vanilla Almond Milk (page 105)

1 cup (128 g) frozen peaches

½ cup (40 g) fresh young coconut meat

1 serving of paleo protein powder

Start by adding the coconut and almond milks to the blender followed by the peaches, coconut meat, and powder.

Blend until smooth.

GUT-BOOSTING TURKEY BURGERS

These turkey burgers provide an added bonus—they are full of flavor but also help support gut health. Coconut oil is a natural antimicrobial that helps keep the pathogenic bacteria in the gut at bay, and probiotic-rich sauerkraut keeps the healthy bacteria in your gut healthy. Pair these burgers with lettuce leaves instead of a bun, and you have yourself a super healthy, easy lunch recipe your digestive health will thank you for!

SERVES 4

1 lb (454 g) organic ground turkey

½ tbsp (7 ml) softened coconut oil, plus extra for cooking

2 cloves garlic, chopped

1 tsp onion powder

½ tsp ground cumin

1 tsp sea salt

¼ tsp black pepper

FOR SERVING

4 tbsp (60 ml) Homemade Paleo-Style Mayonnaise (page 101) (eliminate if following Option 2)

1 avocado, peeled, pitted, and sliced

1 cup (240 g) sauerkraut

Lettuce leaves

Start by adding the ground turkey to a mixing bowl with the ½ tablespoon (7 g) of softened coconut oil, garlic, onion powder, cumin, salt, and pepper. Mix well and then form into 4 burger patties.

Heat a large skillet over medium heat with coconut oil. Cook the burgers for 4 to 5 minutes on each side, or until cooked through.

Serve the burgers with homemade mayonnaise (unless following Option 2), sliced avocado, and sauerkraut on a lettuce leaf.

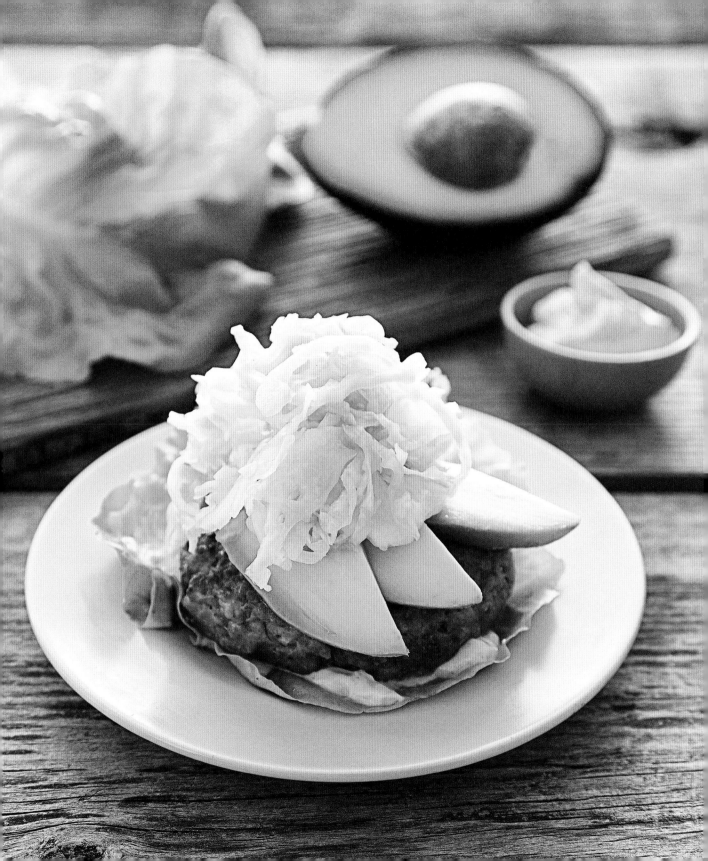

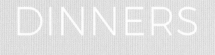

DINNERS

Dinner is my favorite meal of the day, and I tend to add some savory ingredients to my recipes without making preparation too complicated or time-consuming. In this section, I share some of my favorite recipes the whole family will enjoy, including dishes that feature chicken, lamb, beef, bison, liver, and fish.

ROASTED WHITE SWEET POTATOES AND MEATBALLS WITH ROSEMARY AIOLI

This is one of my go-to dinner recipes that the whole family enjoys. The meatballs pair so well with the rosemary aioli sauce, and the roasted white sweet potatoes (page 154) make the perfect side dish. If you love spaghetti and meatballs, try this new healthier variation. It's savory, filling, and full of healthy fat and protein.

SERVES 4

2 tbsp (30 ml) olive oil

1 small yellow onion, chopped

1 lb (454 g) grass-fed ground beef

1 egg (eliminate if following Option 2)

2 cloves garlic, minced

1 tsp sea salt

Pinch of black pepper

1 cup (240 ml) Rosemary Aioli (page 102) (eliminate if following Option 2)

Start by preheating the oven to 350°F (177°C) and lining a baking sheet with parchment paper.

Heat the olive oil in a skillet over medium heat and add the chopped onions. Sauté for 10 minutes, until soft and light brown.

While the onions are cooking, add the ground beef, egg, minced garlic, salt, and pepper to a mixing bowl and stir well to combine.

Once the onions are finished cooking, add them to the meatball mixture and stir to incorporate them into the mixture.

Form the meatball mixture into medium-size meatballs and evenly distribute onto the lined baking sheet.

Bake for 20 to 25 minutes, or until brown and crispy and thoroughly cooked through. Serve with the aioli and roasted sweet potatoes.

(continued)

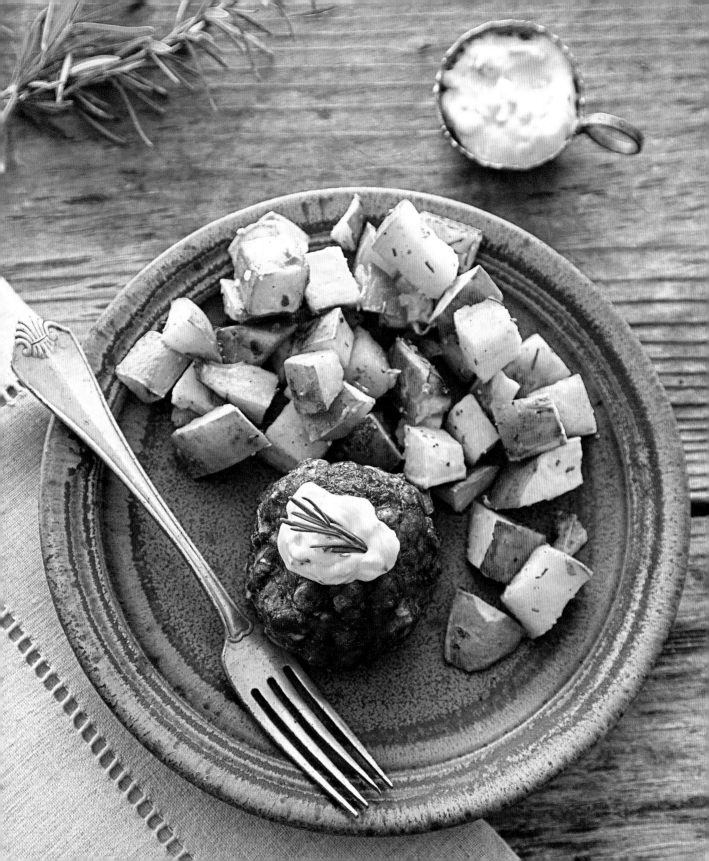

ROASTED WHITE SWEET POTATOES

3 white sweet potatoes, washed and cubed (use regular sweet potatoes if you cannot find white sweet potatoes)

½ small white onion, chopped

2 cloves garlic, minced

¼ tsp sea salt

3 sprigs rosemary, chopped

¼ cup (60 ml) olive oil

Start by preheating the oven to 400°F (204°C) and lining a baking sheet with parchment paper.

Add the potatoes to a mixing bowl and toss with the onion, garlic, salt, rosemary, and olive oil.

Distribute evenly onto the baking sheet and roast for 30 minutes, tossing the potatoes halfway through the cooking time.

Serve with the meatballs and aioli.

ROSEMARY AND GARLIC LAMB CHOPS WITH YUCA FRIES

Many people are intimidated when it comes to cooking lamb chops because they are viewed as a fancy food, but this recipe is so easy to make you could throw it together on a busy weeknight! The garlic and rosemary in this recipe play off one another perfectly. Pair these lamb chops with homemade yuca fries and you have a well-balanced and delicious dinner.

SERVES 4

3 or 4 cloves garlic, minced

4 sprigs rosemary, chopped

½ cup (120 ml) extra virgin light olive oil, plus extra for cooking

Sea salt and pepper to taste

12 grass-fed lamb rib chops

Mix the garlic and rosemary with the olive oil and season with salt and pepper.

Pour the marinade into a resealable bag and add the lamb chops. Shake to thoroughly cover each lamb chop. Refrigerate for 1 hour.

Next, heat a large skillet over medium heat with more olive oil. Add the marinated lamb chops and cook for about 3 minutes on each side, or until cooked to your liking. Serve with the yuca fries.

(continued)

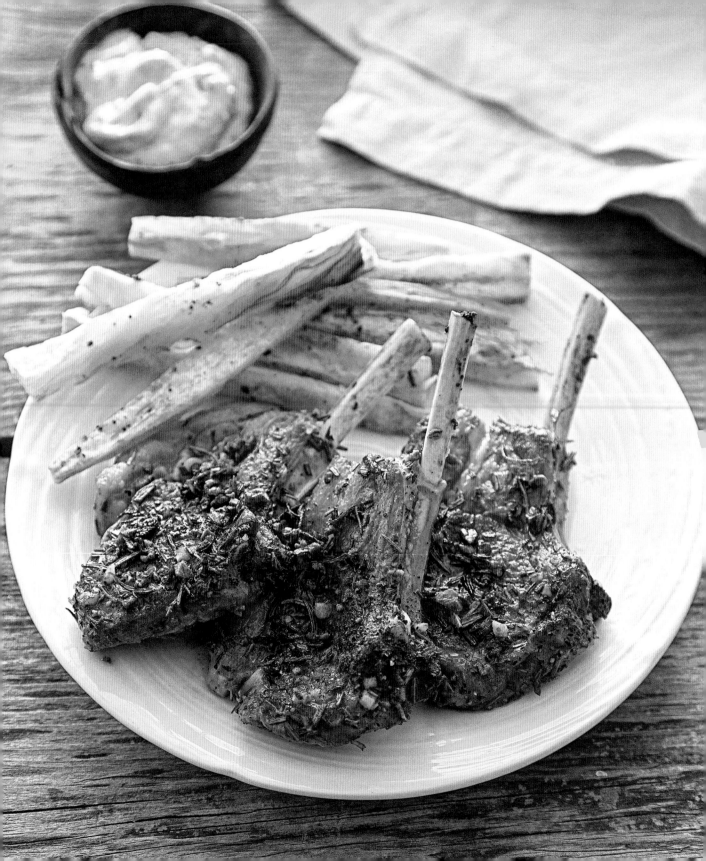

YUCA FRIES

2 yuca roots

¼ cup (60 ml) coconut oil

2 tsp (6 g) garlic powder

Sea salt and pepper to taste

Start by preheating the oven to 450°F (232°C) and lining a baking sheet with parchment paper.

Bring a large pot of water to a boil.

Next, peel the yucas using a vegetable peeler. Cut the yucas in half and then into small french fry shapes.

Use a slotted spoon to carefully add the yuca fries to the pot of boiling water; boil for 10 minutes and then strain.

Next, evenly distribute the fries onto the parchment-lined baking sheet and brush with half the coconut oil and season with the garlic powder, salt, and pepper.

Bake for 12 to 15 minutes, or until lightly brown and then flip and brush with the rest of the oil and bake for another 15 minutes.

Serve with the lamb chops. You may dip them in Rosemary Aioli (page 102) as an option unless you are following Option 2.

SLOW COOKER COCONUT AND LEMON CHICKEN WITH GARLIC AND BASIL CAULIFLOWER RICE

Slow cooker recipes are a lifesaver for anyone who lives a super busy life. You can toss in a handful of nutrient-rich ingredients and let the cooker do all the work for you. This recipe is one of my favorite chicken recipes as it has a mild curry flavor without being too overpowering. It also goes really well with the Garlic and Basil Cauliflower Rice (page 160) instead of white rice, so you can enjoy it without the grains and heavy carbohydrates.

SERVES 4

1 (13.5-oz [398-ml]) can full-fat coconut milk

1 tbsp (6 g) curry powder

½ tsp ground turmeric

½ tsp sea salt

Pinch of ground black pepper

4 chicken breasts

Juice of 1 lemon

2 cloves garlic, minced

1 small yellow onion, diced

Start by whisking together the coconut milk (include the cream), curry, turmeric, salt, and pepper in a medium bowl.

Next, add the chicken breasts to the base of a slow cooker and top with the coconut milk mixture, lemon juice, garlic, and onion.

Cook on low for 6 to 8 hours, or until the chicken is tender and can easily be shredded.

Shred the chicken before serving and enjoy with a side of cauliflower rice (page 160).

(continued)

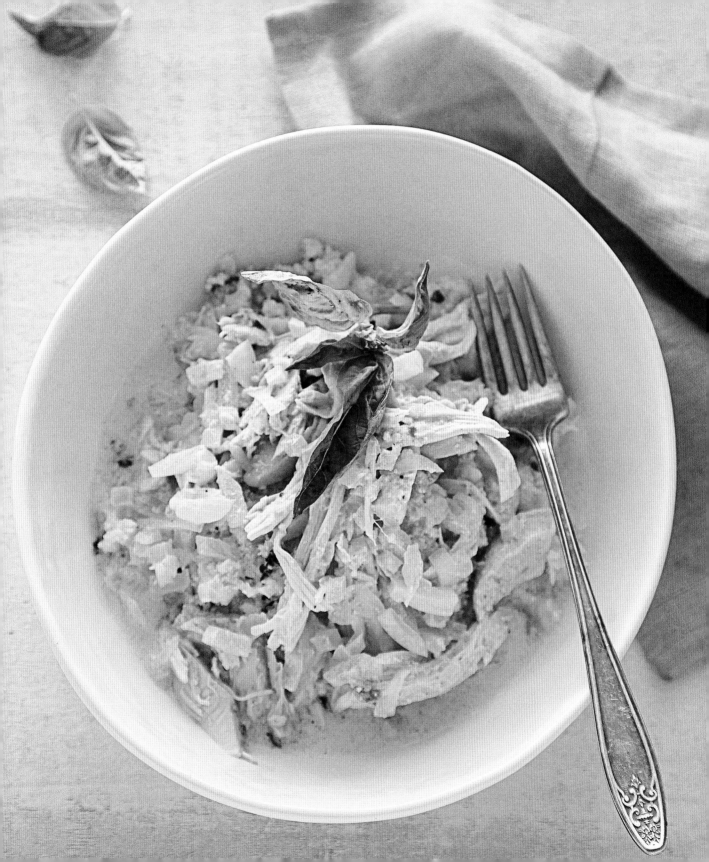

GARLIC AND BASIL CAULIFLOWER RICE

2 heads cauliflower, roughly chopped

2 tbsp (30 ml) olive oil

3 shallots, minced

3 cloves garlic

¾ cup (30 g) chopped basil

Salt and pepper to taste

Start by adding the cauliflower to a food processor, and pulse until it looks like rice.

Preheat a large saucepan with the olive oil. Add the shallots, cook for 5 minutes, then add the garlic and cook for another 2 minutes.

Next, add the cauliflower and continue cooking until it is tender, then add the basil. Season with salt and pepper.

Serve the coconut and lemon chicken over the rice.

BISON BURGERS WITH OVEN-BAKED SWEET POTATO FRIES

Burgers are easy to make, filling, and of course delicious, which is why I have included a couple of different burger variations in this thyroid reset. When made with the right ingredients, burgers can be healthy for you, and this bison burger is no exception. This recipe is full of healthy protein and fat, and pairs well with the Oven-Baked Sweet Potato Fries. This recipe is sure to satisfy your biggest burger and french fry craving!

SERVES 4

1 lb (454 g) ground grass-fed organic bison

2 cloves garlic, chopped

1 tsp sea salt

¼ tsp black pepper

Coconut oil for cooking

FOR TOPPING

8 large lettuce leaves

¼ cup (60 ml) Homemade Paleo-Style Mayonnaise (page 101) (eliminate if following Option 2)

8 tomato slices (eliminate if following Option 2)

1 avocado, peeled, pitted, and sliced

Start by adding the ground bison, garlic, salt, and pepper to a large mixing bowl and mix well to combine. Form into 4 burger patties.

Next, heat a large skillet over medium heat with the coconut oil. Add the burgers and cook for 4 to 5 minutes on each side, until desired doneness.

Serve with lettuce leaves as the bun and top with the mayonnaise, tomato, and avocado and a side of sweet potato fries (page 163).

(continued)

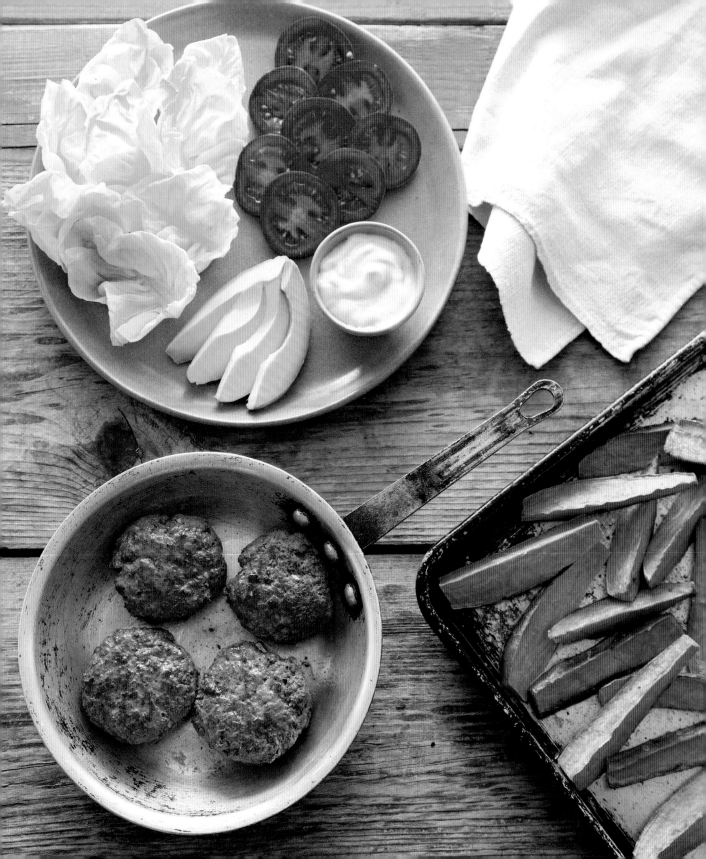

OVEN-BAKED SWEET POTATO FRIES

2 sweet potatoes, peeled and cut into wedges

¼ cup (60 ml) melted coconut oil

1 tsp Himalayan pink sea salt

Start by preheating the oven to 375°F (190°C) and lining a baking sheet with parchment paper.

Evenly distribute the sweet potato wedges onto the sheet and drizzle with the coconut oil. Season with the salt.

Bake for about 30 minutes, or until tender and golden brown, turning them once halfway through the cooking time.

Serve with the bison burgers.

KIMCHI LAMB BURGERS

Here's a delicious lamb burger that puts a healthy spin on the traditional hamburger. The kimchi is packed with probiotics to support a healthy gut, and it also adds a delicious spicy flavor to this recipe. Top with some homemade mayo, and you have a decadent burger that tastes ten times better than any cheeseburger you would get at a restaurant!

SERVES 4

1 lb (454 g) grass-fed ground lamb

2 or 3 cloves garlic, chopped

1 tsp sea salt

¼ tsp ground black pepper

Coconut oil for cooking

8 large lettuce leaves

¼ cup (60 ml) Homemade Paleo-Style Mayonnaise (page 101) (eliminate if following Option 2)

¼ cup (38 g) kimchi (eliminate if following Option 2)

2 handfuls of arugula

Start by adding the ground lamb, garlic, salt, and pepper to a large mixing bowl. Stir well and form into 4 burger patties.

Next, heat a large skillet over medium heat with the coconut oil. Cook the burgers for about 5 minutes on each side, or until cooked to your liking.

Add the cooked lamb burgers to lettuce leaves and smear each burger with 1 tablespoon (15 ml) of mayonnaise. Top with the kimchi and some arugula. Top each burger with another lettuce leaf to form a bun.

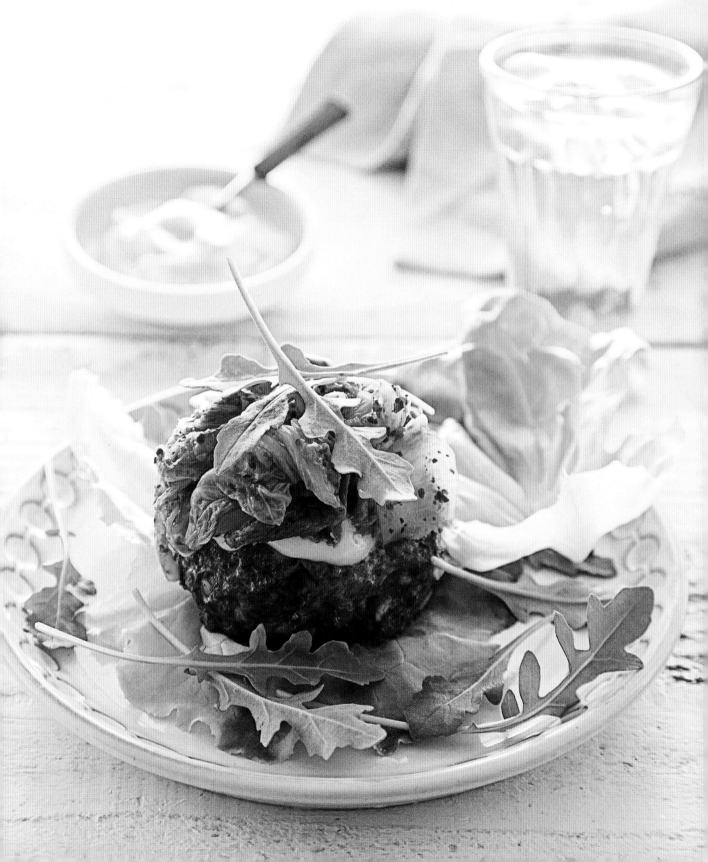

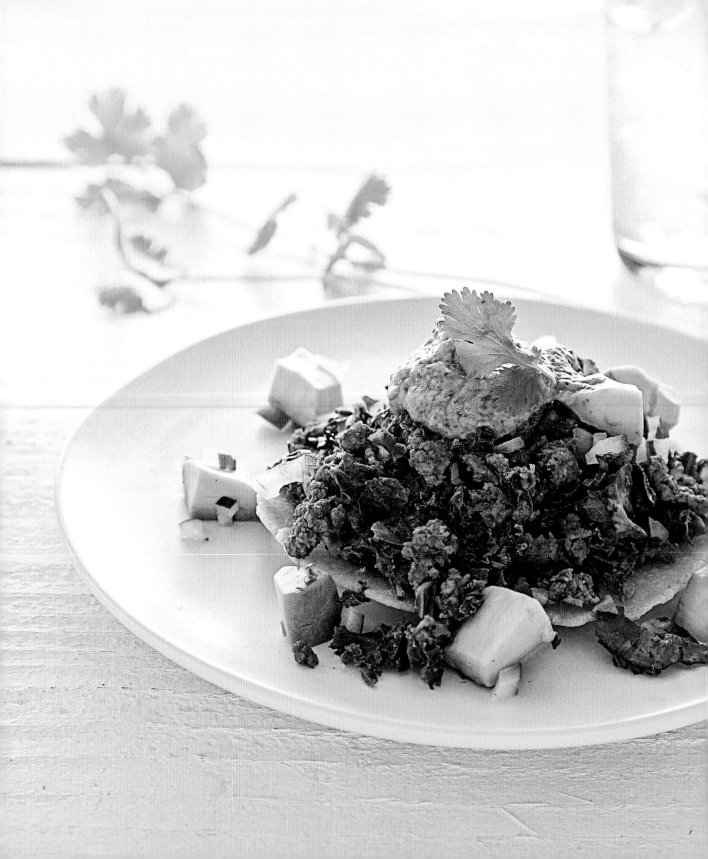

BEEF TACOS

If you love tacos, you are sure to love this beef taco dressed with Green Sauce (page 109). These tacos are a staple in my house because I can easily hide the kale in the recipe without my kids even noticing! This is great for anyone who finds it difficult to get their dark leafy greens in, because the tacos are so bursting with flavor you won't even notice the kale. Pair it with the sauce and you have a delicious and nourishing taco recipe you can enjoy without the guilt.

SERVES 4

Coconut oil for cooking

2 tsp (6 g) ground cumin

1 tsp ground coriander

1 tsp onion powder

1 tsp garlic powder

1 tsp paprika (eliminate if following Option 2 after the initial 30 days)

½ tsp chili powder

1 tsp sea salt

½ tsp ground black pepper

1 lb (454 g) grass-fed ground beef

2 cups (250 g) frozen organic kale

4 to 8 Cassava Tortillas (page 106)

1 recipe Green Sauce (page 109)

Sliced avocado, lettuce, and onion for serving (optional)

Heat a large skillet over medium heat with coconut oil.

While the pan is heating up, add the cumin, coriander, onion and garlic powders, paprika, chili powder, salt, and pepper to a mixing bowl and stir to combine. Set aside.

Add the ground beef to the hot pan and cook until brown, and then add all of the seasoning mix and the kale. Sauté for another 2 minutes and set aside.

Add the cooked ground beef to the center of a tortilla and top with the optional toppings and sauce.

COCONUT-COATED FRIED LIVER WITH ONIONS AND BACON

Chicken liver is something that I recommend my patients eat if they don't mind the flavor. Pair it with bacon and you will forget that you are even eating liver! Liver provides the body with so much nutritional value that it's worth adding to your diet. This is a great recipe to start with, as frying the chicken liver in bacon grease and coating it with spices and coconut flour adds a really nice flavor. If you aren't ready to try chicken liver yet, simply swap the chicken liver for chicken breasts in this recipe.

SERVES 4

1 lb (454 g) organic chicken livers, rinsed and patted dry

¼ cup (28 g) sifted coconut flour

2 tsp (6 g) garlic powder

½ tsp ground coriander

1 tsp sea salt

¼ tsp ground black pepper

4 slices organic nitrate-free bacon, cut into ½" (13-mm) pieces

1 white onion, thinly sliced

1 tbsp (15 ml) coconut oil

Start by chopping the chicken liver into small bite-size pieces.

Next, add the coconut flour, garlic powder, coriander, salt, and pepper to a mixing bowl and whisk to combine.

Dip the chicken liver pieces into the coconut flour mixture to cover both sides and then set aside on a plate.

Next, brown the bacon in a medium frying pan. Remove the bacon using a slotted spoon, leaving the bacon grease in the pan.

Add the chicken livers in a single layer to the bacon grease and fry for 3 to 5 minutes on each side, or until they are crispy.

Set aside on a paper towel to drain off some of the excess oil.

While the chicken livers are cooking, slice the onion, add to another skillet with the coconut oil, and sauté for about 10 minutes or until translucent. Serve with the fried chicken livers and bacon.

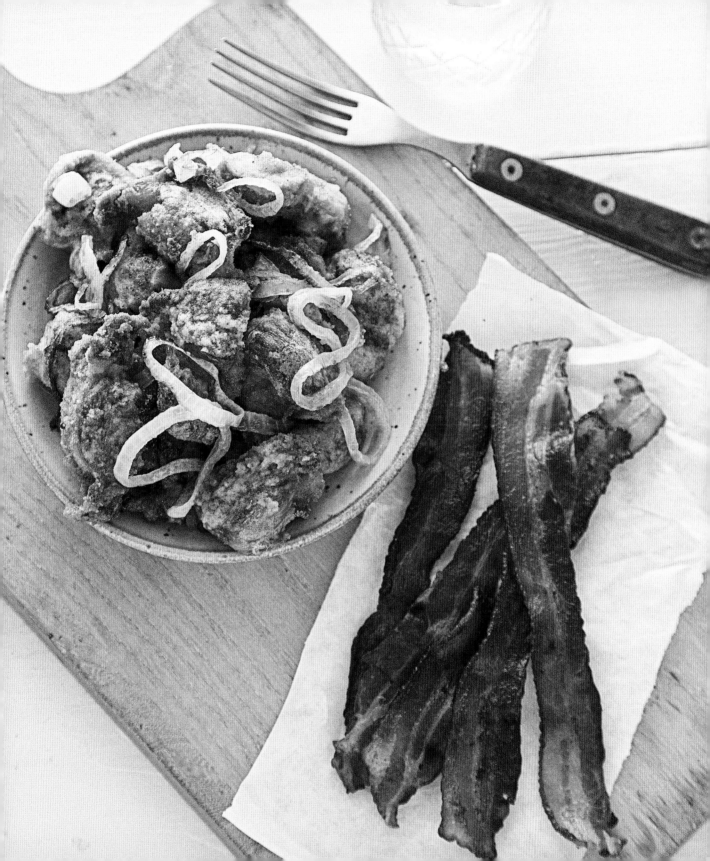

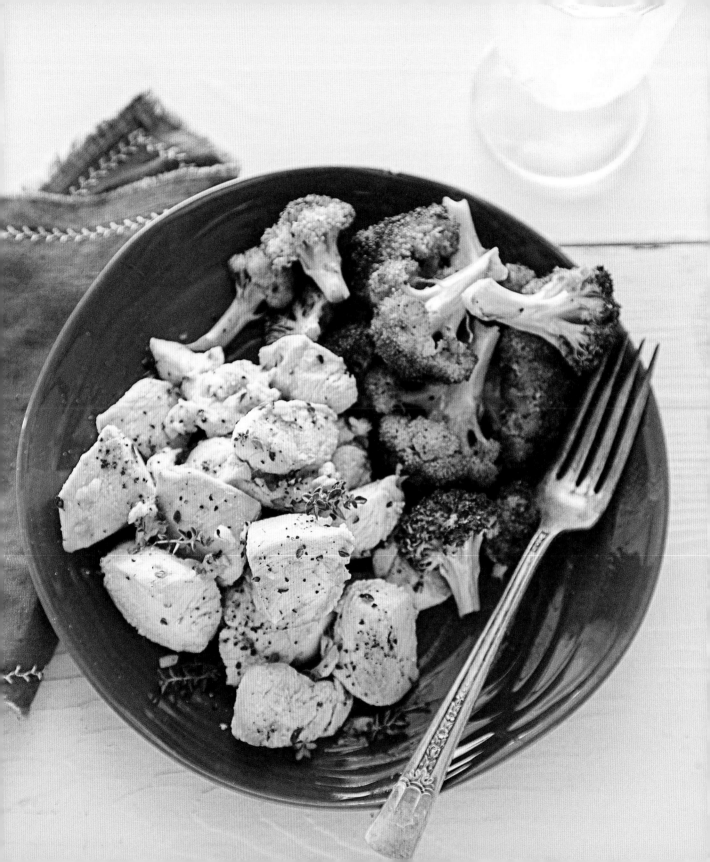

GARLIC CHICKEN WITH BROCCOLI

Chicken breasts make for such an easy weeknight dinner, and while this recipe is super simple to make it doesn't disappoint. Paired with garlic, olive oil, and thyme, this chicken dish has lots of flavor and is something that the whole family will enjoy.

SERVES 4

4 tbsp (60 ml) extra virgin olive oil, divided

4 boneless chicken breasts, cubed

3 cloves garlic, chopped

2 tsp (2 g) chopped fresh thyme

4 cups (360 g) broccoli florets

Sea salt and pepper to taste

Juice of ½ lemon

Heat a large skillet over medium heat with 2 tablespoons (30 ml) of the oil and cook the chicken for about 5 minutes.

Add the garlic and thyme and cook for an additional 5 to 7 minutes, or until the chicken is cooked through.

While the chicken is cooking, preheat the oven to 375°F (190°C) and line a baking sheet with parchment paper.

Evenly distribute the broccoli florets onto the baking sheet. Drizzle with the remaining 2 tablespoons (30 ml) of oil, season with salt and pepper, and roast for about 20 minutes, or until lightly brown.

Serve the cooked chicken with a side of roasted broccoli and a squeeze of lemon juice.

OVEN-ROASTED MACKEREL WITH BRUSSELS SPROUTS

Eating wild-caught fish is such as great way to boost your omega-3 and protein intake. This recipe is a great one for when you want something on the lighter side. It's also paired with roasted Brussels sprouts with bacon, making it an extra savory dish.

SERVES 4

1 lb (454 g) Brussels sprouts, ends trimmed and yellow leaves removed

6 tbsp (90 ml) extra virgin light olive oil, divided

4 slices organic nitrate-free bacon, cut into ½" (13-mm) pieces

4 mackerel fillets, skin on

2 cloves garlic, chopped

1 tsp sea salt

¼ tsp ground black pepper

Lemon juice (optional)

Start by preheating the oven to 400°F (204°C) and lining 2 baking sheets with parchment paper.

Place the Brussels sprouts on the baking sheet and coat with 4 tablespoons (60 ml) of the oil. Add the bacon to the sheet and roast for 30 minutes.

While the sprouts are roasting, season the fillets with the remaining 2 tablespoons (30 ml) of oil, garlic, salt, and pepper and place on the second lined baking sheet skin side up.

Roast the fish for about 10 minutes, or until the fish is completely cooked through.

Drizzle lemon juice over the cooked mackerel if desired and serve with the Brussels sprouts.

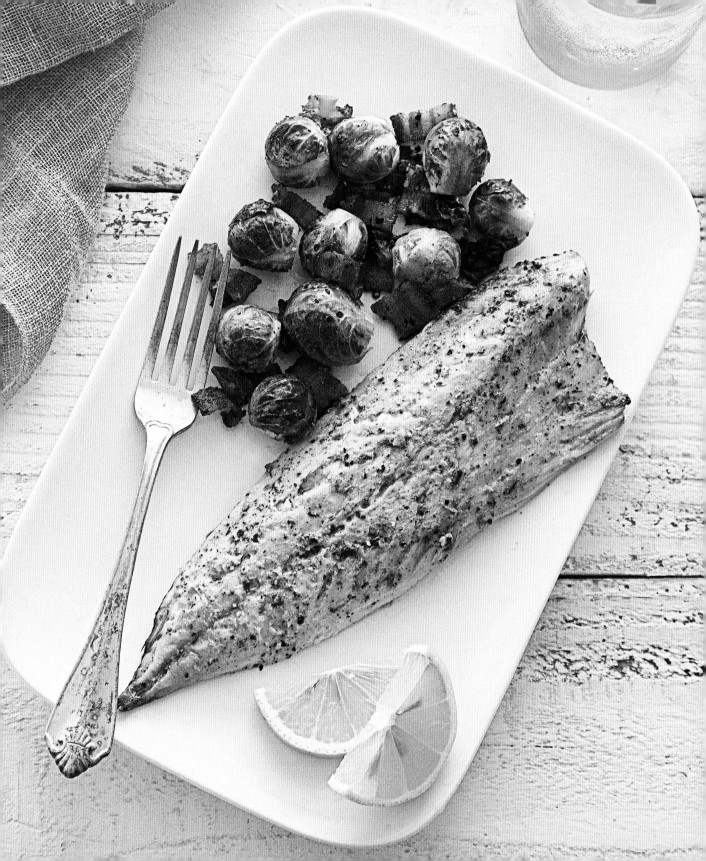

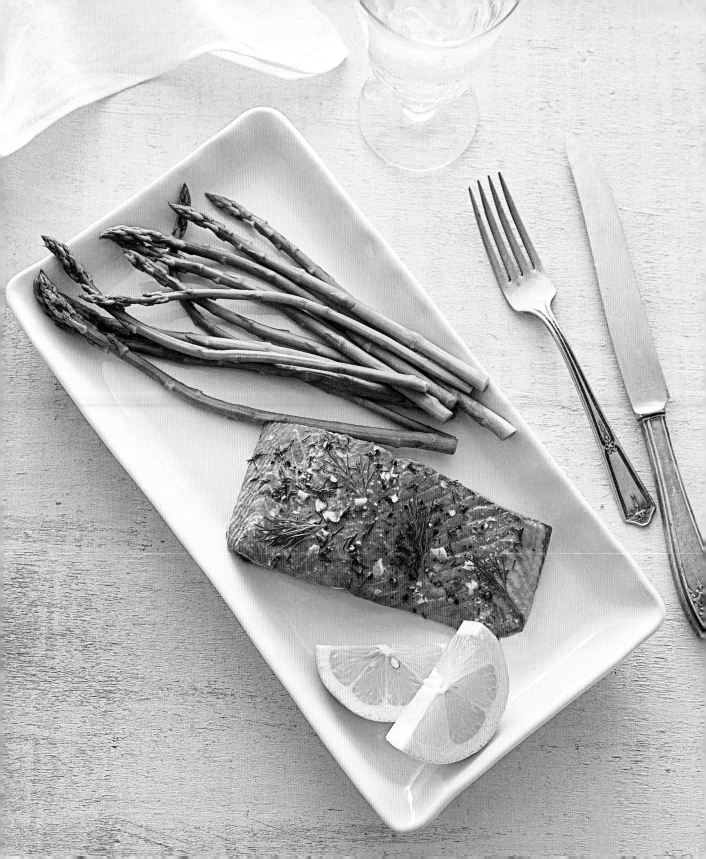

LEMON AND DILL BAKED SALMON WITH ASPARAGUS

As you probably know, salmon is packed full of healthy omega-3 fatty acids to help combat inflammation and boost brain health. Reducing the inflammatory load on your body is an essential step in the reset process, so this recipe makes an excellent addition to your diet. The lemon and dill pair really well together and make for a refreshing light dinner option.

SERVES 4

Coconut oil

4 wild-caught salmon fillets

¼ cup (60 ml) extra virgin light olive oil

¼ cup (60 ml) freshly squeezed lemon juice

1 tbsp (1 g) freshly chopped dill

2 cloves garlic, chopped

Sea salt and pepper to taste

1 bunch asparagus, trimmed

Start by preheating the oven to 350°F (177°C) and greasing a baking dish with coconut oil.

Place the salmon fillets in the baking dish and drizzle with the olive oil and lemon juice. Season with the dill, garlic, salt, and pepper.

Bake for 25 to 30 minutes, or until the fish begins to flake.

While the salmon is baking, bring a large pot of water to a boil, and boil the asparagus for 5 to 7 minutes, or until tender.

Serve the baked salmon with the asparagus.

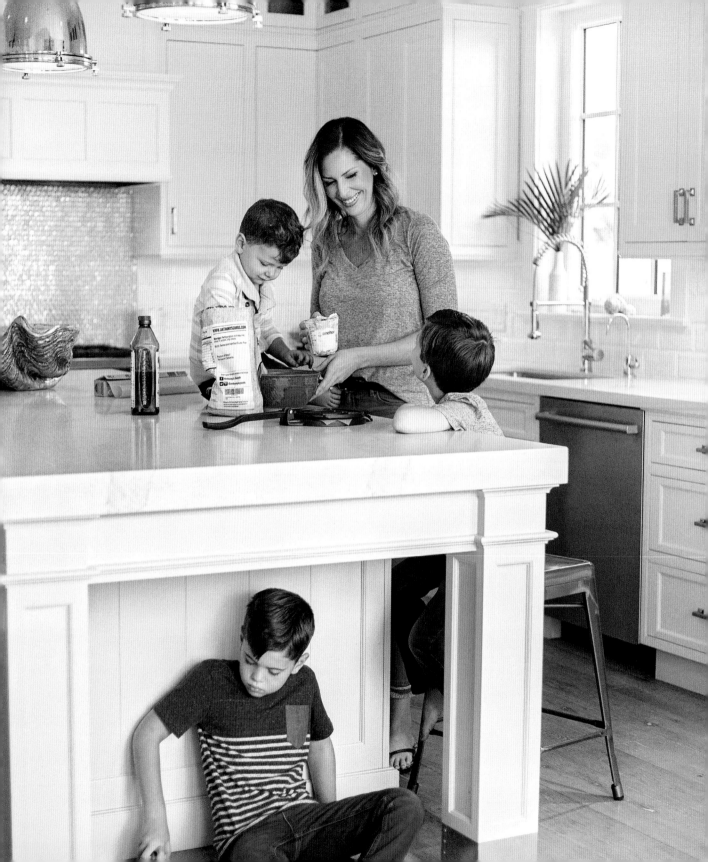

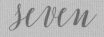

seven

ADDITIONAL
RESOURCES

30-DAY SAMPLE MEAL PLAN

Keep in mind that you can have any breakfast, lunch, or dinner recipe from the thyroid reset that you want; this is just a guide as to what a month on the thyroid reset would look like.

Meal Plan

	DAY 1	DAY 2	DAY 3	DAY 4	DAY 5	DAY 6
BREAKFAST	Breakfast Sausage & Eggs*	Zucchini and Caramelized Onion Scramble*	Pork Patties	Vanilla Chai Smoothie*	Berry Antioxidant Smoothie*	Creamy Avocado Mint Smoothie*
LUNCH	Bone Broth Chicken Soup	Sausage Soup	BLT with Seaweed Salad*	Healthy Egg Salad*	Gut-Boosting Turkey Burgers*	Chicken Salad*
DINNER	Lemon and Dill Baked Salmon with Asparagus	Slow Cooker Coconut and Lemon Chicken wth Garlic and Basil Cauliflower Rice	Bison Burger with Sweet Potato Fries*	Oven-Roasted Mackerel with Brussels Sprouts	Rosemary and Garlic Lamb Chops with Yuca Fries	Roasted White Sweet Potatoes and Meatballs with Rosemary Aioli*

	DAY 7	DAY 8	DAY 9	DAY 10	DAY 11	DAY 12
BREAKFAST	Creamy Berry Smoothie*	Zucchini and Caramelized Onion Scramble*	Sweet Potato Egg Frittata*	Egg Muffins*	Coconut Kefir Parfait	Pork Patties
LUNCH	Wild Salmon Salad*	Sausage Soup	On-the-Go Young Coconut and Peach Lunch Shake*	BLT with Seaweed Salad*	Avocado and Chicken Wrap*	Stuffed Sweet Potatoes with Roasted Garlic Guacamole
DINNER	Beef Tacos*	Slow Cooker Coconut and Lemon Chicken wth Garlic and Basil Cauliflower Rice	Kimchi Lamb Burgers*	Oven-Roasted Mackerel with Brussels Sprouts	Coconut-Coated Fried Liver with Onions and Bacon	Garlic Chicken with Broccoli

	DAY 13	DAY 14	DAY 15	DAY 16	DAY 17	DAY 18
BREAKFAST	Berry Antioxidant Smoothie*	Egg Muffins*	Creamy Berry Smoothie*	Sweet Potato Egg Frittata*	Zucchini and Caramelized Onion Scramble*	Vanilla Chai Smoothie*
LUNCH	Gut-Boosting Turkey Burgers*	Wild Salmon Salad*	Healthy Egg Salad*	Gut-Boosting Turkey Burgers*	Chicken Salad*	Avocado and Chicken Wrap*
DINNER	Roasted White Sweet Potatoes and Meatballs with Rosemary Aioli*	Kimchi Lamb Burgers*	Garlic Chicken with Broccoli	Lemon and Dill Baked Salmon with Asparagus	Roasted White Sweet Potatoes and Meatballs with Rosemary Aioli*	Oven-Roasted Mackerel with Brussels Sprouts

	DAY 19	DAY 20	DAY 21	DAY 22	DAY 23	DAY 24
BREAKFAST	Creamy Avocado Mint Smoothie*	Breakfast Sausage and Eggs*	Breakfast Ground Pork and Plantains	Coconut Kefir Parfait	Berry Antioxidant Smoothie*	Zucchini and Caramelized Onion Scramble*
LUNCH	Stuffed Sweet Potatoes with Roasted Garlic Guacamole	Bone Broth Chicken Soup	Sausage Soup	Wild Salmon Salad*	Chicken Salad*	Gut-Boosting Turkey Burgers*
DINNER	Kimchi Lamb Burgers*	Bison Burger with Sweet Potato Fries*	Slow Cooker Coconut and Lemon Chicken wth Garlic and Basil Cauliflower Rice	Kimchi Lamb Burgers*	Lemon and Dill Baked Salmon with Asparagus	Roasted White Sweet Potatoes and Meatballs with Rosemary Aioli*

	DAY 25	DAY 26	DAY 27	DAY 28	DAY 29	DAY 30
BREAKFAST	Creamy Berry Smoothie*	Creamy Avocado Mint Smoothie*	Egg Muffins*	Zucchini and Caramelized Onion Scramble*	Vanilla Chai Smoothie*	Creamy Avocado Mint Smoothie*
LUNCH	Sausage Soup	Avocado and Chicken Wrap*	Chicken Salad*	Wild Salmon Salad*	Bone Broth Chicken Soup	Healthy Egg Salad*
DINNER	Slow Cooker Coconut and Lemon Chicken wth Garlic and Basil Cauliflower Rice	Beef Tacos*	Coconut-Coated Fried Liver With Onions and Bacon	Kimchi Lamb Burgers*	Roasted White Sweet Potatoes and Meatballs with Rosemary Aioli*	Rosemary and Garlic Lamb Chops with Yuca Fries

30-DAY GROCERY LIST BY WEEK

For week 1, the grocery list will be quite extensive if you do not already have some of the base ingredients such as herbs and spices. Once these are purchased, they will not be repeated on the other weeks' list. For example, coconut oil and dried spices will only be found on week 1—a onetime purchase should get you through the reset. If you have leftover ingredients from the week before, feel free to cross it off the list for the other weeks' list.

Keep in mind that this grocery list was developed assuming that you will make all four servings for each recipe. If you only plan on making one serving per recipe, then the amount you will need to buy will be significantly less. This list is also only for the specific thyroid reset meal plan listed, but remember that you can have any meal in the recipe section that you would like during the thyroid reset. This is just to be used as a guide.

WEEK 1

DAYS 1 TO 7

PRODUCE

- Organic frozen kale
- 1 lb (454 g) Brussels sprouts
- 1 bunch of asparagus
- 2 yuca roots
- 4 yellow onions
- 2 white onions
- 1 Vidalia onion
- 4 green onions
- 3 shallots
- 2 whole heads garlic
- 1 green bell pepper
- 1 bag (10 oz, or 280 g) fresh spinach
- 1 bag (10 oz, or 280 g) arugula
- 1 bunch Swiss chard

- 4 ribs celery
- 1 zucchini
- 1 butternut squash
- 2 heads cauliflower
- 2 sweet potatoes
- 3 white sweet potatoes
- 3 carrots
- 6 tomatoes
- 1 head of lettuce
- 3 bananas
- Frozen mixed berries
- Frozen strawberries
- Frozen blueberries
- 4 green plantains
- 7 avocados
- 1 red apple
- 7 lemons
- Herbs and Spices
- 1 bunch fresh rosemary
- 1 bunch fresh cilantro

- Fresh mint leaves
- Fresh dill
- Fresh basil
- Herbs for bone broth
- Ground coriander
- Paprika
- Curry powder
- Ground cumin
- Ground turmeric
- Chili powder
- Sea salt and pepper
- Ground ginger
- Ground cinnamon
- Ground cloves
- Garlic powder
- Onion powder
- Dried parsley
- Italian seasoning
- Vanilla bean

MEAT, EGGS, SEAFOOD

- 25 eggs
- 1 package (12 oz, or 340 g) organic nitrate-free chicken sausage
- 1 lb (454 g) organic ground pork
- 1 lb (454 g) organic ground turkey
- 12 slices nitrate-free bacon
- 1 package (1 lb, or 454 g) organic nitrate-free Italian sausage
- 8 lb (4 kg) chicken bones for bone broth
- 8 chicken breasts
- 1 whole chicken
- 2 lb (906 g) grass-fed organic ground beef
- 1 lb (454 g) grass-fed organic bison
- 12 grass-fed lamb chops
- 4 wild-caught salmon fillets
- 4 mackerel fillets
- 4 cans (6 oz, or 170 g) wild-caught salmon

FATS AND OILS

- Flaxseeds
- Chia seeds
- Coconut oil
- Extra light tasting olive oil
- Coconut butter

NUTS AND SEEDS

- 1 cup (144 g) almonds

CONDIMENTS

- 2 cans (13.5 oz, or 398 ml) full-fat coconut milk
- Sugar-free Dijon mustard

MISCELLANEOUS

- Coconut wraps
- Cassava flour
- 1 large jar of sauerkraut
- Collagen cleanse powder
- Dried wakame or dulse seaweed
- 1 jar of green olives
- 1 bottle of apple cider vinegar

WEEK 2
DAYS 8 TO 14

PRODUCE

- 1 Vidalia onion
- 4 yellow onions
- 2 white onions
- 1 red onion
- 1 bunch green onions
- 3 whole heads garlic
- 3 shallots
- 1 lb (454 g) Brussels sprouts
- 4 cups (364 g) broccoli florets
- 2 heads cauliflower
- 1 carrot
- 1 zucchini
- 2 ribs celery

- 5 sweet potatoes
- 3 white sweet potatoes
- 1 butternut squash
- 2 bags (10 oz, or 280 g) fresh spinach
- 2 bags (10 oz, or 280 g) fresh arugula
- 1 head lettuce
- Fresh raspberries
- Fresh young coconut meat
- Frozen peaches
- Frozen mixed berries
- 3 green plantains
- 7 avocados
- 5 tomatoes
- 6 lemons
- 1 lime

HERBS AND SPICES

- Fresh oregano
- Fresh thyme
- 1 bunch fresh cilantro
- 1 bunch fresh rosemary
- Fresh basil
- Dried oregano
- Ground coriander
- Herbs of choice for bone broth

MEAT, EGGS, SEAFOOD

- 33 eggs
- 20 strips nitrate-free organic bacon
- 1 lb (454 g) organic ground pork

- 1 lb (454 g) ground organic nitrate-free mild Italian sausage
- 4 lb (1.8 kg) chicken bones for bone broth
- 8 boneless chicken breasts
- 2 organic bone-in chicken breasts
- 2 lb (906) grass-fed organic ground beef
- 1 lb (454 g) organic ground turkey
- 4 cans (6 oz, or 170 g) wild-caught salmon
- 2 lb (906 g) grass-fed ground lamb
- 4 mackerel fillets
- 1 lb (454 g) chicken livers

FATS AND OILS

- Shredded unsweetened coconut
- 3 cans (13.5 oz, or 398 ml) full-fat coconut milk
- Extra light tasting olive oil

NUTS AND SEEDS

- 1 cup (144 g) almonds

MISCELLANEOUS

- Coconut kefir
- Dried wakame or dulse seaweed
- 1 jar of green olives
- Kimchi
- Coconut flour

WEEK 3
DAYS 15 TO 21

PRODUCE

- 3 bananas
- 2 green plantains
- Frozen blueberries
- Frozen strawberries
- 7 sweet potatoes
- 3 white sweet potatoes
- 1 butternut squash
- 8 yellow onions
- 3 white onions
- 1 red onion
- 1 Vidalia onion
- 3 heads garlic
- 3 shallots
- 8 ribs celery
- 3 carrots
- 3 bags (10 oz, or 280 g) fresh spinach
- 1 bag (10 oz, or 280 g) arugula
- 1 head lettuce
- 1 bunch Swiss chard
- 1 bunch asparagus
- 1 zucchini
- 1 green bell pepper
- 2 tomatoes
- 1 lb (454 g) Brussels sprouts
- 4 cups (364 g) broccoli florets
- 2 heads cauliflower

- 1 red apple
- 8 avocados
- 5 lemons
- 1 lime

HERBS AND SPICES

- Fresh oregano
- Fresh basil
- 1 bunch fresh cilantro
- 1 bunch fresh rosemary
- Fresh dill
- Fresh mint leaves
- Herbs for bone broth

MEAT, EGGS, SEAFOOD

- 30 eggs
- 1 package (12 oz, or 340 g) organic nitrate-free chicken sausage
- 4 slices organic nitrate-free bacon
- 1 lb (454 g) ground pork
- 2 lb (906 g) grass-fed organic ground beef
- 1 lb (454 g) grass-fed ground lamb
- 1 lb (454 g) grass-fed organic ground bison
- 1 lb (454 g) organic ground turkey
- 1 whole chicken
- 12 lb (5.5 kg) chicken bones for bone broth
- 2 organic bone-in chicken breasts
- 12 chicken breasts

- 1 lb (454 g) ground nitrate-free organic mild Italian sausage
- 4 wild-caught salmon fillets
- 4 mackerel fillets

NUTS AND SEEDS
- 3 cups (432 g) almonds

MISCELLANEOUS
- 1 can (13.5 oz, or 398 ml) full-fat coconut milk
- Coconut wraps

WEEK 4
DAYS 22 TO 30
PRODUCE
- Fresh raspberries
- Frozen mixed berries
- Frozen blueberries
- Frozen strawberries
- 4 bananas
- 1 green plantain
- 2 Vidalia onions
- 8 yellow onions
- 1 red onion
- 2 white onions
- 3 heads garlic
- 2 ribs celery
- 3 carrots
- 4 white sweet potatoes
- 2 yuca roots
- 1 butternut squash
- 2 zucchini

- 5 avocados
- 3 bags (10 oz, or 280 g) fresh spinach
- 2 bags (10 oz, or 280 g) arugula
- 1 bunch Swiss chard
- 1 head lettuce
- 1 bunch green onions
- 1 bunch asparagus
- 4 tomatoes
- 2 red apples
- 5 lemons
- Frozen organic kale

HERBS AND SPICES
- Fresh mint leaves
- 2 bunches fresh cilantro
- 1 bunch fresh rosemary
- Fresh basil
- Fresh dill
- Fresh herbs of choice for bone broth

MEAT, EGGS, SEAFOOD
- 43 eggs
- 8 strips thick-cut nitrate-free organic bacon
- 8 cans (6 oz, or 170 g) wild-caught salmon
- 2 whole chickens
- 8 chicken breasts
- 1 lb (454 g) chicken livers
- 12 lb (5.5 kg) chicken bones for bone broth
- 1 lb (454 g) organic ground turkey

- 3 lb (1.5 kg) grass-fed ground beef
- 1 lb (454 g) ground organic nitrate-free mild Italian sausage
- 2 organic bone-in chicken breasts
- 2 lb (906 g) grass-fed ground lamb
- 12 grass-fed lamb rib chops
- 4 wild-caught salmon fillets

FATS AND OILS
- Shredded unsweetened coconut
- 2 cans (13.5 oz, or 398 ml) full-fat coconut milk
- Olive oil

NUTS AND SEEDS
- 2 cups (288 g) almonds

MISCELLANEOUS
- Coconut kefir
- 1 jar of green olives
- Coconut wraps

SUPPLEMENTS FOR HASHIMOTO'S

When talking about supplements for Hashimoto's, it's important to understand that supplements aren't meant to take the place of dietary and lifestyle changes. In fact, they are intended to complement all of the wonderful changes that you are making in your life! Adding supplements comes into play when certain vitamin deficiencies may be present, but they always come as a second line of defense to all of the other changes that need to be made when healing from Hashimoto's.

Since the thyroid needs many different nutrients to function at its best, it's important to consume a nutrient-dense diet to try to prevent a deficiency. Some of the nutrients the thyroid needs to work at its best include iodine, selenium, iron, zinc, vitamins A, B2, B12, C, D, and magnesium.

Let's take a look at some of the common supplements used in conjunction with a Hashimoto's healing protocol.

LIVER SUPPORT

Supporting the liver is crucial when supporting your hormones. The liver is an important organ that is responsible for many of our body's processes: it stores glucose for energy, filters the blood, produces and secretes bile for digestion of fat and is one of the places where T4 is converted into T3 (the usable form of thyroid hormone). The liver has an important role in thyroid hormone metabolism and the level of thyroid hormones is also important to normal hepatic function and bilirubin metabolism. You can see why supporting liver function is necessary when supporting thyroid health. On page (194) I share with you the exact supplement and protocol I use to support the liver.

SELENIUM

Selenium is an important nutrient for those with thyroid issues, but it's important to take this nutrient in food form. Getting enough selenium is essential for thyroid function, and it also helps to protect the thyroid from damage from too much iodine exposure. Selenium is also needed for the conversion of T4 into T3. There have been many studies linking the benefits of taking selenium with a thyroid condition. One particular study found that taking selenium had a significant impact on inflammatory activity in thyroid autoimmune disease. When you reduce inflammation, you may also help the body reduce the damage to the thyroid itself. Getting enough selenium in your diet can be as simple as eating two to three Brazil nuts per day, which will add about 200 mcg of selenium! Fish also contains some selenium, so it's good to balance your levels with both high-quality wild-caught fish and Brazil nuts.

I like to recommend getting selenium from food-based sources when possible. If using a supplement, make sure you are using a thyroid-specific blend that has the proper ratio of selenium to iodine like the one I use on page (194). If the iodine to selenium ratio is off balance, it could cause a potential aggravation of hypothyroidism.

IODINE

Iodine is one of the most commonly looked at nutrients when we talk about thyroid health. Iodine is necessary for thyroid hormone synthesis. Some populations, such as women who are of childbearing age, children, vegans, and some pregnant women, may also be at an increased risk for iodine deficiency. Not all supplements or vitamins contain iodine, and iodine intake in the United States has dropped by 50 percent since the 1970s to 1990s according to NHANES data. This could be due to people limiting sources of iodine like dairy, bread, and iodized salt from their diets.

While iodine is often looked at as a key nutrient when talking about thyroid health, we need to talk about the dangers of iodine as well. There have been studies that have shown that an increase in iodine intake, especially in supplement form, may cause an increase in autoimmune attack on the thyroid. The problem with iodine intake when dealing with Hashimoto's often occurs when there is a selenium deficiency present. There was a study done on rats that concluded that the rats that received excess iodine went on to develop goiters. However, when the rats received enough selenium along with the iodine, a goiter did not form. Studies have found that selenium may play a protective role in helping to prevent a flare-up when dealing with autoimmune diseases, which could be caused by excess iodine intake without the addition of selenium. This is why I have a thyroid specific supplement that has the proper ratio of iodine to selenium already measured out on page (194).

VITAMIN C

Vitamin C is a powerful antioxidant and is also excellent for the immune system. Due to the antioxidant content, vitamin C can help protect the thyroid and keep the entire body healthy at the same time.

COD LIVER OIL & VITAMIN D

Cod liver oil is a rich source of vitamins D, A, and E, and DHA and EPA, which are all important when supporting the immune system. Many people don't get enough anti-inflammatory foods from their diet, so supplementing with cod liver oil could help provide your body with the anti-inflammatory benefits your body needs, especially when dealing with an autoimmune condition. Cod liver oil is also known to specifically help lower the risk of autoimmune diseases. For some, cod liver oil will provide enough vitamin D without having to take an additional vitamin D supplement, and others will require both.

CURCUMIN AND RESVERATROL

You may be familiar with resveratrol from the skin of red grapes, and curcumin from the spice turmeric. Both of these compounds contain incredibly powerful antioxidant and anti-inflammatory properties. These two are particularly unique because when used together they have shown to have some powerful effects against Hashimoto's disease. While both of these compounds are powerful on their own, studies have shown that taking them together creates a synergistic effect. This is especially useful for anyone dealing with an autoimmune condition or anyone who is suffering from a significant amount of inflammation. Without getting too technical, there is some science behind why this powerful combo works so well against autoimmune diseases such as Hashimoto's.

There is a specific immune pathway in autoimmunity and inflammation called TH-17. This pathway helps fight off viruses and bacteria. However, overstimulation of TH-17 can cause autoimmune flare-ups and lead to inflammation. When curcumin and resveratrol are used together, they have been shown to help reduce the activation of TH-17, which will ultimately help protect the tissue from further damage in cases of autoimmunity. Curcumin and resveratrol have also been shown to help support regulatory T cells, which are cells that regulate the immune system. When regulatory T cells do not work the way that they should, the immune system can trigger Hashimoto's flare-ups.

PROBIOTICS

Probiotics are important for gut health, and part of supporting Hashimoto's means taking care of the digestive system (remember, most people with autoimmune conditions also suffer from a leaky gut). The majority of our immune system also resides in the gut, which is another very important reason to consume foods and supplement when necessary to help our gut work the way it should.

Probiotics are great for promoting the healthy bacteria in the GI tract, and I always recommend soil-based or spore-based probiotics a soil-based product that provides the body with resilient microflora and helps mimic the natural flora that was once found in Paleolithic diets. A spore-based probiotic supplement that is designed to survive in the gastric system and then colonize to provide the desired effects you would look for in a high-quality probiotic supplement. The spores also work to defend and protect the gut from harmful microbes, help support the immune system, and improve digestion, to name a few of the amazing benefits.

However, before any probiotic supplementation recommendations are made, I always like to test for gut infections, as this helps provide the best direction in terms of the appropriate supplement for you.

IRON

A deficiency in iron can lead to problems with thyroid hormone production. An iron deficiency reduces heme-dependent thyroid peroxidase activity in the thyroid. However, too much iron can damage the hypothalamus, pituitary, and thyroid gland. In fact, too much iron can be so damaging that it can cause an 80 times greater chance of developing hypothyroidism according to a study. So what does this mean? This means that we want to have adequate levels of iron in the body for our thyroid to function at its best, but we also want to be careful not to overdo it and cause even further damage to thyroid health. Working with a functional medicine practitioner is an important step in making sure your iron levels are where they need to be. It may also be best to focus on iron-rich foods instead of iron supplements in many cases to avoid iron toxicity. Some great food sources of iron include oysters, clams, liver, venison, and beef.

ZINC

Zinc is an essential trace element with numerous benefits for the body, like supporting our immune system and establishing hormone balance. Zinc may be one of the most essential elements in thyroid function as it is essential for healthy levels of T3 (triiodothyronine). Zinc also plays an essential role in the conversion of T4 to T3 and increasing levels of T4 and T3. Zinc is also included in my thyroid-specific supplement on page (194).

THYROID MEDICATION

As I mentioned throughout the book, while some people may be able to catch thyroid disease before medication is needed, this is not the case for everyone. There are times where there is just too much damage and medication is 100 percent necessary. I wanted to expand on thyroid medications so that you can better understand the importance of taking it if needed and also cases where medication may not be entirely necessary.

Let's start with the overmedication dilemma we commonly experience in the United States. Many doctors prescribe drugs as a quick fix, but the problem is that medications do not get to the root of the problem. Medications may put a band-aid on the problem, but they will not provide a permanent cure. Many patients are put on thyroid medications right away, even if their T3 and T4 levels are not depleted. There was a study published in *Internal Medicine* that found that a very common thyroid medication levothyroxine had very little benefit when prescribed to those with borderline hypothyroidism. Prescribing thyroid medications to someone who may be suffering from a borderline thyroid condition and not a total depletion may not sound like such a bad thing, but these drugs can come with pretty significant side effects.

In cases where medication is not truly needed, patients may not get any benefit from the medication at all and could ultimately suffer side effects, like irregular heart rhythms, insomnia, and even a loss of bone density. The truth is that thyroid medications are being overprescribed and dietary, lifestyle, and even appropriate supplementation could manage the borderline condition while also getting to the root cause. Prescriptions of levothyroxine skyrocketed to 70 million in 2010! Here's one more reason why it's so important to work with a skilled professional who has extensive experience in thyroid health. The last thing you want is to be prescribed a medication that may do absolutely nothing for you but cause unwanted symptoms and still not get to the bottom of what's causing the imbalance to begin with.

In cases where thyroid medication is given before T3 and T4 levels are depleted, it's likely that these patients do not need the medications and could go on without ever needing them with the right dietary and lifestyle changes. I work with many patients who come to me with borderline thyroid conditions and through investigating what's causing the imbalance in their body they are able to restore health and stop the condition from developing into a full-blown autoimmune thyroid disease.

The major issue comes in when your thyroid has been under attack for too long, and you already have too much damage to the tissues. In cases like this, you absolutely must take your thyroid medication because, as you now know, the thyroid provides essential hormones that affect every single cell in your body. If you ignore the issues and don't take your medication when there is major damage, you risk putting your health at stake, and the outcome could be debilitating.

If you have been prescribed medication or are wondering which option may be best for you, here are some thyroid medication options. These are desiccated thyroid brands, and there are quite a few options. Knowing a little bit about each is important as you can speak with your doctor about which option may be best for you before he or she prescribes something. Here are two options you may be interested in speaking with your doctor about if you do need to take medication.

NATURETHROID

This desiccated thyroid medication has been around since the 1930s and has since been reformulated. Many patients are happy with taking this particular brand. Below you will find the current ingredient list for Naturethyroid.

- Colloidal silicon dioxide
- Dicalcium phosphate
- Lactose monohydrate
- Magnesium stearate
- Microcrystalline cellulose
- Croscarmellose sodium
- Stearic acid
- Opadry II 85F19316 clear
- Porcine thyroid powder, U.S. pharmacopeia (USP)

WP THYROID

WP Thyroid is another popular thyroid medication that has been around for quite some time. Westhroid was around before Westhroid-P, which came on the market in 2013 and which many patients have been happy with. This is because there are only two listed fillers—inulin from chicory root and medium-chain triglycerides from coconuts. It's also important to note that there is lactose in this prescription medication. RLC Labs notes that this particular medication is gluten free. According to RLC labs, here is what this drug consists of:

- T4 and T3 replacement hormones (desiccated porcine thyroid)
- Thyroid cofactors (T1, T2, calcitonin, and iodine) naturally occur in trace amounts

REPAIRING GUT HEALTH

The bottom line about medication is that at times it's necessary, but that's not the case for everyone with Hashimoto's disease. If we can find the root cause and the triggers of Hashimoto's, then we can get the body to stop attacking itself. For some people, this means total remission and no need for medication, ever. For other people, this means that they will have to stay on their medication but can keep the condition from getting worse and get rid of most if not all of their symptoms. In my practice, I work with both kinds of patients. No matter what the case, I always emphasize the importance of gut health, as this is where the majority of the immune system is and with Hashimoto's disease, we are dealing with an autoimmune condition. Once we work on building and repairing the gut, we move on to other healing protocols to support the thyroid while also getting to the root of what's causing the thyroid problem to begin with.

It's important to understand that while everyone would like to be medication–free, having to stay on your medication doesn't disqualify you from making massive strides in your health and preventing your condition from getting worse. So, if you do have to continue to take your medication, do not be discouraged. There is so much good you can do for your body that will ultimately help improve your health for the long run.

MEAL PREP FOR SUCCESS

Let's face it: meal prepping can be a chore, especially when you don't have a specific plan in place. The truth is that if you do some meal prep each week, you will set yourself up for a path of success when it comes to your eating habits. A large part of healing from Hashimoto's involves dietary changes, so you will want to focus a lot of attention on what you are putting into your body.

If meal preparation is not something you look forward to, I have some tips to make it a little more enjoyable and less like a chore.

COOK IN MULTIPLE BATCHES: When you are making a recipe, make multiple batches. Freeze what you aren't going to use right away and then have meals to enjoy later. This will save you lots of time.

PREP YOUR SNACKS: Snacks are tough for a lot of people. When you get hungry in between meals, it's easy to just consume anything that's available, but those options may not be the healthiest choices. Instead, prep your snacks so you always have something fresh and readily available. Make some batches of homemade trail mix with nuts, dried fruit, and some seeds, and cut up some fresh fruit to enjoy. If you have some snacks that need to be refrigerated, be sure to put them in the front of your fridge so that they are easy to just grab and go and you are more likely to make the healthier choice.

STOCK UP ON STORAGE CONTAINERS: Storage containers are a must when you are meal prepping, and I recommend you buy the glass options to avoid any BPA or BPS exposure. You can find some inexpensive options online, so stock up when you see a good deal. You will be using these a lot when meal prepping!

PORTION OUT YOUR LUNCHES: If lunch is one of the hardest meals of the day for you, you may want to portion out your meals. Now, chances are meal prepping just one day a week isn't going to get you through the entire week, so you will need to set aside some time a few days a week. Maybe you spend Sundays prepping Monday through Wednesday's meals, and then you put some time aside on Wednesday prepping the rest of the week. No matter how you do it, cooking some chicken, turkey, grass-fed beef, and steamed veggies ahead of time and portioning them into lunch sizes is a great way to stay on top of your healthy eating throughout the week.

WASH AND PREP PRODUCE AHEAD OF TIME: Once you get home from the store or farmers' market, you will save yourself so much time if you wash your produce right away. This will make things so much easier for you during the week when you just want to grab and go or take some veggies out of the fridge and prep a recipe. You can even make your own homemade fruit and vegetable wash with water and vinegar.

SLOW COOKER: Super busy? Make the slow cooker your best friend. You can make so many nutritious meals in a slow cooker, so search for recipes you think you may like to make that are paleo friendly and try them out. When you find ones you like the most, make more than one batch at a time to freeze for later use when you are too busy to cook on a weeknight.

PREP SALADS IN A CANNING JAR: If you usually have a salad for lunch, you can prep your salad the night before in a convenient on-the-go canning jar. This makes things really easy when it comes to packing your lunch in the morning for work.

PREP YOUR MORNING SMOOTHIES: If you have smoothies in the morning, why not make it super easy on yourself by getting all the ingredients ready to go the night before? You can put them in a freezer-safe glass container to just toss in the blender before you head out to work.

SHOP ACCORDING TO YOUR NEEDS: Some people only like to go to the store once per week, while others find it more convenient to go a couple of times per week. Find out what works for your schedule and stick to it. This will help ensure you always have healthy food available, and you will be less likely to order takeout.

MAKE A MEAL PLAN: Making a weekly or monthly meal plan is one of the best ways to stay on top of your healthy eating and a great way to make meal prepping easier. You will know what you are going to eat when, and you can plan ahead. This will also make grocery shopping a whole lot easier!

Meal prepping can take some getting used to, especially if you have been eating out or just whipping up whatever you have available. By putting a little time into your weekly meal plans, you can be meal prepping like a pro in no time. This is an integral part of the healing journey, so be sure to implement some of these tips to make sticking to your meal plan easier and more enjoyable.

HELPFUL TRACKING TOOLS

In the modern world, electronics are able to track everything, and they can serve as very useful tools when we are trying to stay on track with our diet and exercise routines. Here are some of my favorite apps and other tracking methods that I commonly recommend to my patients.

DR. CAMPBELL'S FAVORITE DIET AND EXERCISE TRACKERS

I love these online and phone apps and trackers as a way to help patients track their food intake and exercise. They are also very useful for goal setting, and you are even able to look up specific nutritional information about certain foods.

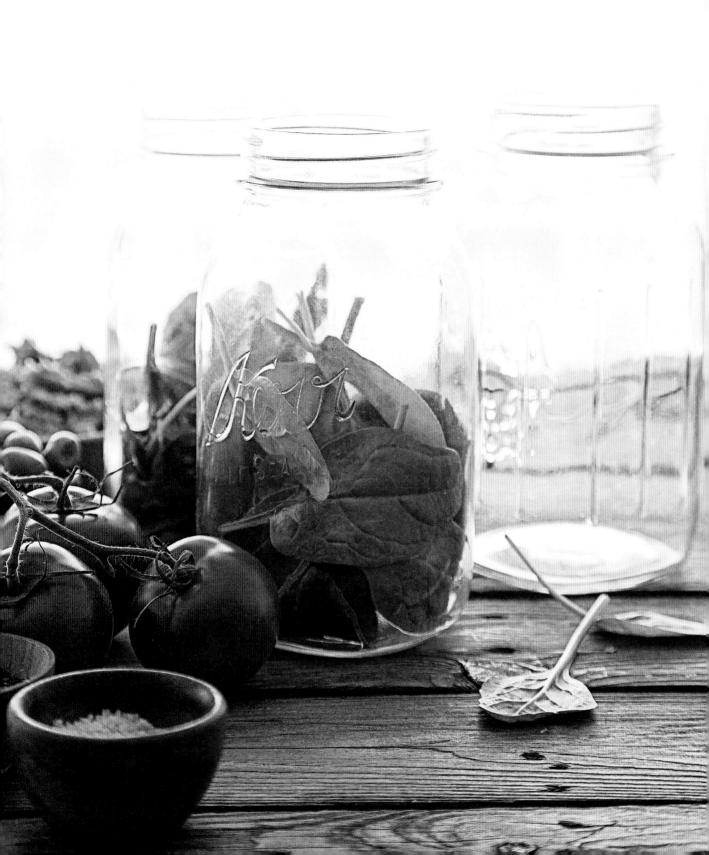

FATSECRET: Diet tracker

MYFITNESSPAL: Diet tracker

FITBIT: A great fitness tracker that can also help monitor heart rate, water intake, and sleep patterns.

MAPMYFITNESS: This fitness tracker provides running maps as well as workouts that you can use in the gym, and you can keep track through their mobile app on your phone.

STRONGLIFTS: This is an app that provides you with 45-minute workouts if you need some motivation on how to get started with your exercise routine.

JAWBONE UP: Similar to the Fitbit with a wristband and progress tracking app. You can track things like sleep as well as activity and dietary intake.

SLEEP TRACKERS

Just as diet and exercise are important parts of the Hashimoto's healing protocol, sleep is essential as well. For my patients who have irregular sleep patterns or just struggle with getting enough sleep, I recommend that they track their sleep. Here are some of my favorite sleep trackers.

SLEEP CYCLE: This is an excellent app that tracks your sleep pattern and then wakes you up during a period of light sleep within a certain set time period. It helps you wake up more naturally than the standard alarm clock.

DEEP SLEEP: This is a great app for anyone who has a difficult time falling asleep at night. It's a guided meditation app that is specifically designed to help you get to sleep faster.

STRESS-BUSTING APPS

Stress is another element of the Hashimoto's healing protocol. You need to tackle autoimmune disease from every angle, and addressing stress levels is part of the equation. Many of my patients find it helpful to have a stress-management app available to help with reminders and to track their progress each day. Here are some of my personal favorite stress-management apps.

HEADSPACE: This app provides guided meditations that you can do during a break from work or in the middle of the day when you just need a timeout. It's also great if you are new to meditation and need some help getting into a routine.

CALM: Another guided meditation app that slowly introduces the practice of meditation and is very easy to follow.

YOUTUBE YOGA VIDEOS: I love to recommend yoga to many of my patients for stress reduction. It's a free and gentle way to calm the body and the mind, and there are so many free videos online you can access from the comfort of your own home. Try a couple until you find one that you enjoy most and stick to it.

I am always adding new recipes, videos, and blog posts at www.drbeckycampbell.com, or DrBeckyCampbell on Facebook, drbeckycampbell on Instagram, and on my YouTube channel.

DR. CAMPBELL'S FAVORITE NATURAL PRODUCTS

BEAUTYCOUNTER: I love ordering my skin care products and makeup from Beautycounter. They offer safer products that are much better for our skin than products you would purchase in stores. It is so important that we look at the products we are using on our skin, as the skin is the largest organ in the body. What we choose to put on our skin matters, as the skin absorbs the toxins from the products we are using. Unfortunately, there are countless toxins used in skin care and makeup products and each of these toxins has the potential to cause disruption in the body. This is the last thing you want when you are trying to reset your body and promote thyroid health. Taking care of our body is more than just watching the foods we consume; it's also about what we use on our skin every day. This is why I am so selective about the products I use. You can take a look at Beautycounter and what they have to offer by visiting https://www.beautycounter.com/beckycampbell1.

YOUNG LIVING ESSENTIAL OILS: I recommend the use of essential oils to many of my patients. Not only do they smell amazing, but they also hold some health benefits. Essential oils are a great substitute for anyone who is used to wearing perfume or scented lotion, or likes to use air fresheners in their home. Essential oils can take the place of all three of these things in a much safer and healthier way. You can use essential oils in a diffuser throughout your home, add essential oils to unscented lotions to make your own scented lotion free from chemicals, and mix oils with coconut oil to use as a healthy alternative to perfume. Essential oils have been used for thousands of years for their medicinal properties, and some have the ability to promote relaxation. Each oil holds a different benefit, and some have even been shown to hold antibacterial properties and even digestive health benefits. Some of my favorite essential oils are lavender for relaxation, and Endoflex by Young Living Essential Oils for endocrine system support. Visit Young Living at http://yl.pe/3298.

DR. CAMPBELL'S THYROID SUPPORT SUPPLEMENT GUIDE

This is the exact supplement protocol I use during the first 30 days along with the diet in this book with my patients.

WEEKS: 1–4

OPTIMAL RESET PALEO PROTEIN SHAKE: 2 SHAKES PER DAY

This is a nutrient-dense meal supplement with a low glycemic impact, nutrients in their bioidentical forms, healthy fats and complete hydroBEEF bone broth protein isolate sourced from animals raised without hormones and fed a diet free from GMO grains, grasses and hay. This is great to use as a complement to a low-calorie meal or alone as a snack. It comes in chocolate and vanilla flavors and can be found on my website store (drbeckycampbell.com/shop/).

OPTIMAL RESET LIVER LOVE: 2 CAPSULES, TWICE PER DAY

This is a synergistic formula designed to support healthy liver function. With a blend of mushroom and botanical extracts, plus N-Acetyl-L-Cysteine (NAC), which has powerful antioxidant and liver-supporting actions. NAC also assists with the formation of glutathione, which is the main predominant antioxidant found in the liver.

AFTER WEEKS 1–4:

Discontinue the Optimal Reset Liver Love supplement and reduce the Optimal Reset Paleo Protein Shake to 1 shake per day. Then add:

OPTIMAL RESET ULTIMATE THYROID SUPPORT: 2 CAPSULES PER DAY

This all-in-one formula was designed to support the ultimate function of the thyroid gland. This blend helps maintain healthy cortisol, blood glucose and insulin levels, along with a balanced conversion of thyroid hormone and essential vitamins and minerals that the thyroid needs.

For more information about what tests you need and a more specific plan to discover your hidden triggers, check out my Optimal Thyroid Reset Program on my website. In this program, I offer specific tools to uncover what tests you need, links to order those tests and a comprehensive guide for each test, plus specific supplement protocols to discover what your body needs to fully recover.

REFERENCES

CHAPTER 1

Beyer, Edward. Thyroid Recovery. Thyroid Success Secret #1: Your lab ranges are too wide! http://thyroidrecoverydocs.com/thyroid-success-secret-1-your-lab-ranges-are-too-wide.htm.

Gutner, Marina. Why Thyroid Tests Can be Tricky. http://outsmartdisease.com/tsh-normal-range-and-normal-thyroid-levels.

Hashimoto's Disease. National Institutes of Health. https://www.niddk.nih.gov/health-information/endocrine-diseases/hashimotos-disease.

Kresser, Chris. HPA-D:Etiology. Adapt Framework Level 1, kresserinstitute.com.

Lanzisera, Frank. The Six Systems and Organs Affected by Thyroid Disease. *Total Health Magazine*. www.totalhealthmagazine.com/Thyroid-Health/The-6-Main-Systems-and-Organs-Affected-by-Thyroid-Disease.html.

Milas, Kresimira. Hashimoto's Thyroiditis Overview. Endocrine Web. https://www.endocrineweb.com/conditions/hashimotos-thyroiditis/hashimotos-thyroiditis-overview.

Toft, Daniel J. Graves' Disease Overview. Endocrine Web. https://www.endocrineweb.com/conditions/graves-disease/graves-disease-overview.

CHAPTER 2

Gallagher, CM, and JR Meliker. Mercury and thyroid autoantibodies in U.S. women, NHANES 2007–2008. PubMed. https://www.ncbi.nlm.nih.gov/pubmed/22280926.

Goop. The Medical Medium. http://goop.com/the-medical-medium-and-whats-potentially-at-the-root-of-medical-mysteries.

Greenfield, B. Two Ways Your Brain Breaks and Exactly What You Can Do About It Part 2. https://bengreenfieldfitness.com/2013/08/how-to-fix-hpa-axis-dysfunction.

Gutner, Marina. How Estrogen Dominance Can Ruin Your Thyroid Health. Outsmart Disease. http://outsmartdisease.com/how-estrogen-dominance-can-ruin-your-thyroid-health.

Kresser, Chris. HPA-D: Etiology. Adapt Framework Level 1, kresserinstitute.com.

——. Iodine for Hypothyroidism: Crucial Nutrient or Harmful Toxin? https://chriskresser.com/iodine-for-hypothyroidism-like-gasoline-on-a-fire.

——. The Role of Vitamin D Deficiency in Thyroid Disorders. https://chriskresser.com/the-role-of-vitamin-d-deficiency-in-thyroid-disorders.

——. Selenium: The Missing Link for Treating Hypothyroidism? https://chriskresser.com/selenium-the-missing-link-for-treating-hypothyroidism.

——. The Thyroid-Gut Connection. https://chriskresser.com/the-thyroid-gut-connection.

National Institute of General Medical Sciences. Circadian Rhythms Fact Sheet. https://www.nigms.nih.gov/Education/Pages/Factsheet_CircadianRhythms.aspx.

Sterzl, I, J Prochazkova, P Hrda, P Matucha, J Bartova, and V Stejskal. Removal of dental amalgam decreases anti-TPO and anti-Tg autoantibodies in patients with autoimmune thyroiditis. *Neuroendocrinology Letters*. Dec 2006. https://www.ncbi.nlm.nih.gov/pubmed/16804512.

Tamer G, S Arik, I Tamer, and D Coksert. Relative Vitamin D Insufficiency in Hashimoto's Thyroiditis. *Thyroid*. Aug 2011. https://www.ncbi.nlm.nih.gov/pubmed/21751884.

Wentz, Izabella. Blood Sugar Imbalances and Hashimoto's. https://thyroidpharmacist.com/articles/blood-sugar-imbalances-and-hashimotos.

——. Food Sensitivities and Hashimoto's. http://thyroidpharmacist.com/articles/food-sensitivities-and-hashimotos.

CHAPTER 3

Axe, Josh. The Hypothyroidism Diet. https://draxe.com/hypothyroidism-diet-natural-treatment.

Ballantyne, Sarah. T*he Paleo Approach. Reverse Autoimmune Disease and Heal Your Body*. Victory Belt Publishing, 2014.

Cohen, Suzy. 14 Essential Oils for a Healthy Thyroid. http://suzycohen.com/articles/essential-oils-thyroid-health.

Endocrine Web. How Stress Affects Your Thyroid. https://www.endocrineweb.com/conditions/thyroid/how-stress-affects-your-thyroid?page=1.

Kresser, Chris. 9 Steps to Perfect Health. https://chriskresser.com/9-steps-to-perfect-health-8-sleep-more-deeply.

———. HPA-D:Etiology. Adapt Framework Level 1, kresserinstitute.com.

———. Why You May Need to Exercise Less. https://chriskresser.com/why-you-may-need-to-exercise-less.

Mindful. Getting Started with Mindfulness. http://www.mindful.org/meditation/mindfulness-getting-started.

Natural Endocrine Solutions. Exercise and Thyroid Health. http://www.naturalendocrinesolutions.com/articles/exercise-thyroid-health.

Wheeler, Mark. Sleepless Nights Triggers Immune System's Inflammatory Response. http://newsroom.ucla.edu/releases/Sleepless-Night-Triggers-Immune-7335.

CHAPTER 4

Body Ecology. Getting to the Root of Autoimmune Disorders. http://bodyecology.com/articles/getting-to-the-root-of-autoimmune-disorders-anemia-food-sensitivity-and-more.

Gallagher, C, and J Meliker. Mercury and Thyroid Autoantibodies in U.S. Women, NHANES 2007–2008. *Environment International* volume 40 (April 2012). http://www.sciencedirect.com/science/article/pii/S0160412011002716.

Health Line. Food Allergy vs. Sensitivity: What's the Difference? https://www.healthline.com/health/allergies/food-allergy-sensitivity-difference.

Myers, Amy. The Toxin, Heavy Metal, and Thyroid Connection. http://www.amymyersmd.com/2015/07/the-toxin-heavy-metal-and-thyroid-connection.

Schoenfeld, Laura. 5 Steps to Personalizing Your Autoimmune Paleo Protocol. https://chriskresser.com/5-steps-to-personalizing-your-autoimmune-paleo-protocol.

CHAPTER 7

Axe, Josh. 11 Benefits of Cod Liver Oil. https://draxe.com/cod-liver-oil.

———. Top 10 Foods High in Selenium. https://draxe.com/top-10-foods-high-selenium.

Endocrine Web. Thyroid Gland, How It Functions, Symptoms of Hyperthyroidism and Hypothyroidism. https://www.endocrineweb.com/conditions/thyroid-nodules/thyroid-gland-controls-bodys-metabolism-how-it-works-symptoms-hyperthyroid.

Functional Health News. Combine Resveratrol and Curcumin to Quench Hashimoto's Flare Ups. http://functionalhealthnews.com/2014/10/resveratrol-curcumin-inflammation-autoimmune-2.

Get Real About Hypothyroidism. Natural Hypothyroidism Treatment. http://getrealthyroid.com/why-get-real/wp-thyroid.

Godman, Heidi. For Borderline Underactive Thyroid, Drug Therapy Isn't Always Necessary. http://www.health.harvard.edu/blog/for-borderline-underactive-thyroid-drug-therapy-isnt-always-necessary-201310096740.

Guilliams, T. *The Role of Stress and the HPA Axis in Chronic Disease Management*. Point Institute, 2015.

Health Line. Autoimmune Diseases: Types, Symptoms, Causes and More. http://www.healthline.com/health/autoimmune-disorders.

Huang MJ1, Liaw YF. "Clinical associations between thyroid and liver diseases." *Journal of gastroenterology and hepatology* 1995 May-Jun;10(3):344-50. Pub Med. Web. 19 Oct. 2018

Kresser, Chris. HPA-D: Etiology. Adapt Framework Level 1, kresserinstitute.com

———. Selenium: The Missing Link for Treating Hypothyroidism? https://chriskresser.com/selenium-the-missing-link-for-treating-hypothyroidism.

Mayo Clinic. Hashimoto's disease. http://www.mayoclinic.org/diseases-conditions/hashimotos-disease/symptoms-causes/dxc-20269764.

Moducare. https://www.moducare.com.

Osanksy, Eric M. The Relationship Between Natural Progesterone and Thyroid Health. Thyroid Nation. http://thyroidnation.com/natural-progesterone-thyroid.

Prescript Assist. http://www.prescript-assist.com/products.

Stop the Thyroid Madness. Armour vs Other Brands. https://stopthethyroidmadness.com/armour-vs-other-brands.

WebMD. Hashimoto's Thyroiditis. http://www.webmd.com/women/hashimotos-thyroiditis-symptoms-causes-treatments.

Wentz, Izabella. Going Dairy Free to Reverse Hashimoto's. http://thyroidpharmacist.com/articles/going-dairy-free-to-reverse-hashimotos.

ACKNOWLEDGMENTS

I want to acknowledge my patients and my followers, who have put their trust in my programs and become a part of a community. I thank you all for your endless support.

Thank you to everyone at Page Street for having faith in my work and turning my manuscript into a beautiful book.

ABOUT THE AUTHOR

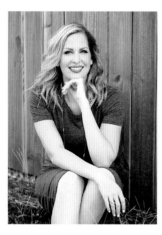

DR. BECKY CAMPBELL is a board-certified doctor of natural medicine (DNM) and a doctor of chiropractic (DC). She is the creator of the Optimal Reset Plan and founder of DrBeckyCampbell.com. She has worked for the last ten years to try to help others find the root cause of their thyroid disease and hopes this book will guide readers to optimal health.

WORKING WITH ME

Are you ready to get the testing you need and start a protocol designed just for you? Many clients come to me when they want to get to the bottom of what may be going on. Here are some other reasons patients choose to work with a functional medicine practitioner:

- You don't want to rely on unnecessary drugs and medical intervention for the rest of your life.
- You are interested in discovering the underlying cause of your problems, rather than just suppressing symptoms.
- You are motivated to play an active role in your own healing process
- You are willing to make the necessary dietary and lifestyle changes to support health and well-being.

HOW DO I WORK WITH PATIENTS?

One way to think of functional medicine practitioners is as health detectives. We focus on identifying and addressing the underlying cause of an illness, rather than just suppressing symptoms.

Like all detectives, we use a variety of tools in our investigations, including detailed questionnaires, a thorough medical history and examination, and comprehensive laboratory tests (blood, urine, stool, breath, hair testing, and more).

We then use nutritional therapy, herbal medicine, supplements, stress management, detoxification, lifestyle changes, and—in some cases and only when necessary—prescription medications to eliminate triggers and restore proper function and balance.

Deep and lasting healing is only possible when the root causes of illness are addressed. By understanding the core systems of the body, how they are related, and how their function can be restored, many chronic illnesses can be prevented and even reversed.

WHAT IS MY TREATMENT PHILOSOPHY?

I practice a new model of medicine, sometimes referred to as functional or systems medicine. Functional medicine is neither conventional nor alternative medicine. It's a combination of the best elements of both, and it represents the future of medicine.

WHAT CONDITIONS DO I SPECIALIZE IN?

I have particular experience with and training in:

- Digestive problems and food intolerances
- Thyroid conditions
- Low immune function, allergies, asthma
- Autoimmune disease
- Hormone imbalances (adrenal, thyroid, sex hormones)
- High cholesterol
- Fatigue, low energy, poor sleep
- Cognitive and neurological disorders

If you're ready to get started, contact me at https://drbeckycampbell.com.

INDEX